H

D1615984

Curing
Depression
Naturally

with
Chinese
Medicine

C4

Rosa N. Schnyer
& Bob Flaws

BLUE POPPY PRESS

Published by:
BLUE POPPY PRESS, INC.
3450 Penrose Place, Suite 110
BOULDER, CO 80301

First Edition, July, 1998
ISBN 0-936185-94-5 LC 97-77990
COPYRIGHT 1998 © BLUE POPPY PRESS

COMP Designation: Original work and functionally translated compilation

Printed at Johnson Printing in Boulder, CO
on essentially chlorine-free paper
Cover design by Jeff Fuller, Crescent Moon
10 9 8 7 6 5 4 3 2 1

Other books in this series include:
Curing Insomnia Naturally with Chinese Medicine
Curing Hay Fever Naturally with Chinese Medicine
Breast Health Naturally with Chinese Medicine
Curing Depression Naturally with Chinese Medicine
Curing Arthritis Naturally with Chinese Medicine
Curing PMS Naturally with Chinese Medicine

Preface

Depression seems to be epidemic in our society. Every day, we meet people who are currently on antidepressants. On the one hand, the discovery of a new line of medications, such as Zoloft and Prozac, has made antidepressants easily administered, and, therefore, *also over-prescribed*. On the other hand, the rapidly growing demands of our cultural evolution submit us to very high levels of physical and emotional stress. We find ourselves depleted of inner resources, struggling to catch up.

Depression affects people's lives in profound ways. It touches every aspect of the human experience—our physical well-being, our relationships with our loved ones, our work, our creativity, our spirituality. Depression can paralyze and alienate us, making us strangers to ourselves and the world we inhabit.

As an acupuncturist and practitioner of Chinese medicine involved in research funded by the National Institutes of Health (NIH), I have had the opportunity to assist numerous people suffering from depression. I have seen Chinese medicine help transform hopelessness into possibility, helplessness into courage, anxiety into calmness. Therefore, with the help of Bob Flaws, I have written this book as a comprehensive guide for laypersons to the treatment of depression with Chinese medicine. It presents an overview of the fundamental principles which underlie the theory and practice of acupuncture and Chinese herbal medicine, *and* it instructs the reader on preventive techniques, numerous home remedies, and information on how to create an individualized regime.

We live in a society accustomed to avoiding pain, which refuses delayed gratification and resists any change that requires effort.

The idea of altering our mood and escaping the complexity of a depressive episode quickly and effortlessly is quite appealing. Our tendency to reduce biological and psychological processes to mechanistic interactions reinforces the treatment of depression as a linear event. If there is a deficit of neurotransmitters such as serotonin, then making more serotonin available should resolve depression. There is no doubt that antidepressants are sometimes indispensable and life-saving for many people. However, these drugs fail to address the more complex chain of interactions, both biological and psychological, which typically contribute to depression.

Currently, there is a new wave of enthusiasm to replace antidepressant drugs with botanical extracts, for example, St Johnswort (Hypericum perforatum). St. Johnswort has been widely tested in Europe in the treatment of mild to moderate depression. While this natural approach has clear advantages over conventional drugs (it has no known side effects!), it fails to treat the person as a whole and still approaches depression as a separate entity separate from the person.

Chinese medicine offers an alternative and complementary approach to the understanding and treatment of depression. It aims at integrating body and mind. It too is free of side effects. And it empowers the person to make changes in their life. With this book, we hope to make the wealth of information on the Chinese medical treatment of this devastating disease widely available to readers in the West. We also hope that it contributes to eradicating the stigma associated with psychological distress and mental illness in general.

Rosa N. Schnyer
Tucson, AZ,
October 1997

Table of Contents

Introduction

Joan was feeling increasingly irritable and frustrated. She wanted to hide and not see people and she had no desire to do anything at all. She had lost interest in life and felt apathetic. She was tired all the time and spent long periods of time staring at the wall. Even though she was always exhausted, she felt restless and anxious. She fidgeted constantly when sitting at her desk performing her job which she hated. She had gained quite a bit of weight because she felt constantly hungry. Food calmed her down, but it also made her sluggish and bloated. Often she would burst out crying over any little thing and she had difficulty sleeping through the night. Her dreams were vivid and disturbing.

If this story sounds familiar, this book may help you overcome the cycle of depression. Traditional Chinese doctors have treated the symptoms of depression safely and effective for tens of centuries.

This book is a layperson's guide to the diagnosis and treatment of depression. In it, you will learn what causes depression *and what you can do about it*. Hopefully, you will be able to identify yourself and your symptoms in these pages. If you can see yourself in the signs and symptoms we discuss below, we feel confident that we will be able to share with you a number of self-help techniques which can minimize your discomfort. I (RS) have been a professional practitioner of Chinese medicine for over 10 years, and I have helped numerous Western patients cure, relieve, or manage their depression. Chinese medicine cannot cure every disease, but when it comes to a depressive episode,

Chinese medicine is an invaluable alternative. Not only is Chinese medicine very effective for curing or at least reducing the symptoms of depression, if you follow the advice presented in this book, you can also help prevent the recurrence of depressive episodes. Long-term, chronic depression and depression complicated by other factors can also be addressed by Chinese medicine. Chinese medicine may not totally cure these more complicated and recalcitrant types of depression, but it can greatly help reduce their symptoms and teach you how to manage your condition.

What is depression?

According to the DSM-IV, the *Diagnostic and Statistical Manual of Mental Disorders*, 4th edition, depression is a type of mood disorder which is not due to any organic factor. It is characterized by a depressed mood or loss of interest and is typically accompanied by several other associated symptoms. Here we are not talking about psychotic disorders which may also affect one's mood, such as schizophrenia, schizoaffective disorder, or delusional disorder. And we are also not talking depression alternating with manic episodes (*i.e.,* the predominance of an elevated mood). Depression which does not include manic episodes is called unipolar depression, while depression alternating with manic episodes is called bipolar disorder. A mild and persistent type of bipolar disorder is known as cyclothymia.

Types of depression

There are a number of types of depression according to Western psychiatry/psychology. Since your Western clinician may have diagnosed you with one of these terms, it is useful to know what they mean. Let's begin with the two main types of depression: major depression and dysthymia. The main difference between these two is that dysthymia refers to low-grade, chronic depression, while major depression refers to an acute depressive episode. In many cases, major depressive episodes may occur to those already suffering from low-grade, chronic depression. This is then called double depression. Major depression is also subdivided into mild, moderate, or severe grades, and the severe grade may occur with or without such psychotic features as delusions or hallucinations. If a current depressive episode has lasted two consecutive years without a period of two months or longer in which there were no depressive symptoms, this is called chronic depression. If the onset of recurrent depression has a regular cyclic relationship with a particular period of the year (for example, if one always feels depressed when winter begins and feels completely better when spring arrives), this is called seasonal pattern depression.

Major depression

The essential features of a major depressive episode are a depressed or irritable mood or loss of interest or pleasure in all or most activities for at least two weeks in a row. A person is diagnosed as being depressed if A) no organic cause can be found which started and maintained the depression and B) if the depressed mood is not the normal reaction to the loss of a loved one. Some symptoms associated with depression include either increased or loss of appetite, lack of energy, increased desire to sleep or an inability to fall and/or stay asleep, a feeling of worthlessness or excessive and inappropriate guilt, difficulty concentrating, and possible recurrent thoughts of death or suicide. A person experiencing depression may also be unable to sit still or may feel "slowed down." The smallest tasks seem difficult and require a long time to complete. One may also feel tearful and anxious, ruminate obsessively, and be overly concerned with one's physical health.

Dysthymia

Also called depressive neurosis, dysthymia is a chronic condition that involves a depressed mood (or possible irritability in children and adolescents) that has lasted for at least two years (or one year for children or adolescents). Additional symptoms may include sleep disturbance and appetite changes. During this period, the person is never without depressive symptoms for more than two months. To clinically diagnose dysthymia, there must not have been a major depressive episode at the onset of the disturbance or a history of a chronic psychotic condition.

Frequently, dysthymia appears to be the consequence of a chronic non-mood disorder, such as anxiety, anorexia, substance dependency, or rheumatoid arthritis. In this case, it is called secondary dysthymia. When it doesn't appear to be related to a pre-existing chronic disorder, it is called primary dysthymia.

A milder, yet more prevalent form of depression

Interestlingly, a recent study headed by Dr. Louis Judd, former director of the National Institutes of Mental Health, found that many people who do not meet the current diagnostic criteria for depression, nevertheless, suffer from a real impairment due to one or more symptoms of this illness. Many times, such sufferers lack the symptoms of a depressed mood. This milder depression is four times more prevalent than clinical depression. The three most common symptoms reported in this case are fatigue, sleep disturbance, and thoughts of death. Dr. Judd calls this condition "subsyndromal symptomatic depression."[1]

Causes of depression

For years Western clinicians and researchers have debated whether depression is essentially biological or psychological in nature. Most likely it is both. Some people seem to be vulnerable to a biological imbalance. However, this vulnerability is usually triggered by specific life events which are processed psychologically. At the same time, psychological factors seem to

---

[1]   Micheal, Norden J., *Beyond Prozac*, Harper Collins Publishers Inc., NY, 1995, p. 7

precipitate a complex series of biological symptoms which are part of the experience of depression. So, as with many things in life, it is not so easy to say that depression is "all in your head" or all in your genes. Rather, the truth probably lies somewhere within the complex interactions of "nature and nurture."

How Western medicine treats depression

Western medicine emphasizes pharmacotherapy or psycho-therapy as its two main therapies in the treatment of depression. Pharmacotherapy means the administration of internal medicines. It is based on the biological perspective of depression. Basically, it involves the prescription of antidepressants. There are three main types of antidepressants: monoamine oxidase (MAO) inhibitors, tricyclic antidepressants (TCA's), and selective serotonin re-uptake inhibitors (SSRI's). This last group, the SSRI's, are currently the most commonly used and include Prozac, Zoloft, and Paxel. Unfortunately, antidepressants have a wide range of side effects. For example, if MAO inhibitors are taken in combination with a diet that includes chocolate, oranges, cheese, and other foods which contain large amounts of tyramine, they can cause high blood pressure. The side effects caused by the tricyclics are not as dangerous, but they are quite unpleasant nonetheless. These include drowsiness, blurred vision, consti-pation, and a dry mouth. The SSRI's like Prozac can cause headache, anxiety, upset stomach, and decreased libido or sexual desire. They can also cause agitation, violence, and thoughts of suicide in a small number of people.

The psychotherapeutic treatment of depression includes three main approaches. There is the psychodynamic approach, the humanistic-existential approach, and the cognitive-behavioral approach. Each of these approaches emphasizes a different theory of the causation of depression. We won't go into the details of these different theories here. However, for further information on these three types of psychotherapeutic approaches to depression, interested readers should see the bibliography. In terms of psychotherapy, Cognitive Behavioral Therapy (CBT) is currently considered one of the most effective approaches to the treatment of depression, while the medical standard of care is to combine the use of antidepressants with short-term psychotherapy.

Both the pharmacological and psychotherapeutic approaches alleviate depression in 50-70% of people who complete treatment. Nevertheless, both treatments fail to provide lasting relief for a sizable number of depressed persons. In addition, a significant number of people terminate therapy prior to its completion. Further, depression tends to be a chronic, recurrent disorder. Even when it is successfully treated with either Western drugs or psychotherapy, depression tends to recur. This is why there is a consensus among those who treat depression that some form of continued maintenance treatment is necessary after initial recovery has occurred.

Fortunately, Chinese medicine offers safe, effective, low cost alternatives for the treatment of depression which have been used in Asia for hundreds and thousands of years. Chinese medicine not only has a good record of success, it has no side effects when correctly administered, it is preventive, and it addresses both the body and mind. In fact, as we will see below, there is no division between the body and mind in Chinese medicine. In addition, Chinese medicine empowers patients to make changes in their lives and participate in their own health recuperation and maintenance.

East is East and West is West

In order for the reader to understand and make sense of the rest of this book on Chinese medicine and depression, one must understand that Chinese medicine is a distinct and separate system of medical thought and practice from modern Western medicine. This means that one must shift models of reality when it comes to thinking about Chinese medicine. It has taken the

Chinese more than 2,000 years to develop this medical system. In fact, Chinese medicine is the oldest continually practiced, literate, professional medicine in the world. As such one cannot understand Chinese medicine by trying to explain it in Western scientific or medical terms.

Most people reading this book have probably taken high school biology back when they were sophomores. Whether we recognize it or not, most of us Westerners think of what we learned about the human body in high school as "the really real" description of reality, not one possible description. However, if Chinese medicine is to make any sense to Westerners at all, one must be able to entertain the notion that there are potentially other valid descriptions of the human body, its functions, health, and disease. In grappling with this fundamentally important issue, it is useful to think about the concepts of a map and the terrain it describes.

If we take the United States of America as an example, we can have numerous different maps of this country's land mass. One map might show population. Another might show per capita incomes. Another might show religious or ethnic distributions. Yet another might be a road map. And still another might be a map showing political, *i.e.*, state boundaries. In fact, there could be an infinite number of potentially different maps of the United States depending on what one was trying to show and do. As long as the map is based on accurate information and has been created with self-consistent logic, then one map is not necessarily more correct than another. The issue is to use the right map for what you are trying to do. If one wants to drive from Chicago to Washington, D.C., then a road map is probably the right one *for that job* but is not necessarily a truer or "more real" description of the United States than a map showing annual rainfall.

What we are getting at here is that *the map is not the terrain*. The Western biological map of the human body is only one potentially useful medical map. It is no more true than the

7

traditional Chinese medical map, and the "facts" of one map cannot be reduced to the criteria or standards of another *unless they share the same logic right from the beginning*. As long as the Western medical map is capable of solving a person's disease in a cost-effective, time-efficient manner without side effects or iatrogenesis (meaning doctor-caused disease), then it is a useful map. Chinese medicine needs to be judged in the same way. The Chinese medical map of health and disease is just as "real" as the Western biological map as long as, using it, professional practitioners and their patients are able to solve their patients' health problems in a safe and effective way.

Therefore, the following chapter is an introduction to the basics of Chinese medicine. Unless one understands some of the fundamental theories and "facts" of Chinese medicine, one will not be able to understand or accept the reasons for some of the Chinese medical treatments of depression. As the reader will quickly see from this brief overview of Chinese medicine, "This doesn't look like Kansas, Toto!"

An Overview of the Chinese Medical Map

In this chapter, we will look at an overview of Chinese medicine. In particular, we will discuss yin and yang, qi and blood, essence and spirit, the viscera and bowels, and the channels and network vessels. In the following chapter, we will also look at the concept of qi stagnation and the relationship of both the menstrual cycle and aging to this concept of qi stagnation. Once we understand these things, we can then go on to see how Chinese medicine views depression and how professional practitioners of Chinese medicine diagnose and treat the various patterns of depression.

Yin & Yang

To understand Chinese medicine, one must first understand the concepts of yin and yang since these are the most basic concepts in this system. Yin and yang are the cornerstones for understanding, diagnosing, and treating the body and mind in Chinese medicine. In a sense, all the other theories and concepts of Chinese medicine are nothing other than an elaboration of yin and yang. Most people have probably already heard of yin and yang but may have only a fuzzy idea of what these terms mean.

The concepts of yin and yang can be used to describe everything that exists in the universe, including all the parts and functions of the body. Originally, yin referred to the shady side of a hill and yang to the sunny side of the hill. Since sunshine and shade are two, interdependent sides of a single reality, these two aspects of the hill are seen as part of a single whole. Other examples of yin and yang are that night exists only in relation to day and cold exists only in relation to heat. According to Chinese thought, every single thing that exists in the universe has these two aspects, a yin and a yang. Thus everything has a front and a back, a top and a bottom, a left and a right, and a beginning and an end. However, a thing is yin or yang *only in relation to its paired complement*. Nothing is in itself yin or yang.

It is the concepts of yin and yang which make Chinese medicine a holistic medicine. This is because, based on this unitary and complementary vision of reality, no body part or body function is viewed as separate or isolated from the whole person. The table below shows a partial list of yin and yang pairs as they apply to

Yin	Yang
form	function
organs	bowels
blood	qi
inside	outside
front of body	back of body
right side	left side
lower body	upper body
cool, cold	warm, hot
stillness	activity, movement

the body. However, it is important to remember that each item listed is either yin or yang only in relation to its complementary partner. Nothing is absolutely and all by itself either yin or yang. As we can see from the above list, it is possible to describe every aspect of the body in terms of yin and yang.

10

Qi

Qi (pronounced chee) and blood are the two most important complementary pairs of yin and yang within the human body. It is said that, in the world, yin and yang are water and fire, but in the human body, yin and yang are blood and qi. Qi is yang in relation to blood which is yin. Qi is often translated as energy and certainly energy is a manifestation of qi. Chinese language scholars would say, however, that qi is larger than any single type of energy described by modern Western science. Paul Unschuld, perhaps the greatest living sinologist, translates the word qi as influences. This conveys the sense that qi is what is responsible for change and movement. Thus, within Chinese medicine, qi is that which motivates all movement and transformation or change.

In Chinese medicine, qi is defined as having five specific functions:

1. Defense
It is qi which is responsible for protecting the exterior of the body from invasion by external pathogens. This qi, called defensive qi, flows through the exterior portion of the body.

2. Transformation
Qi transforms substances so that they can be utilized by the body. An example of this function is the transformation of the food we eat into nutrients to nourish the body, thus producing more qi and blood.

3. Warming
Qi, being relatively yang, is inherently warm and one of the main functions of the qi is to warm the entire body, both inside and out. If this warming function of the qi is weak, cold may cause the flow of qi and blood to be congealed similar to cold's effect on water producing ice.

11

4. Restraint

It is qi which holds all the organs and substances in their proper place. Thus all the organs, blood, and fluids need qi to keep them from falling or leaking out of their specific pathways. If this function of the qi is weak, then problems like uterine prolapse, easy bruising, or urinary incontinence may occur.

5. Transportation

Qi provides the motivating force for all transportation and movement in the body. Every aspect of the body that moves is moved by the qi. Hence the qi moves the blood and body fluids throughout the body. It moves food through the stomach and blood through the vessels.

Blood

In Chinese medicine, blood refers to the red fluid that flows through our vessels the same as in modern Western medicine, but it also has meanings and implications which are different from those in modern Western medicine. Most basically, blood is that substance which nourishes and moistens all the body tissues. Without blood, no body tissue can function properly. In addition, when blood is insufficient or scanty, tissue becomes dry and withers.

Qi and blood are closely interrelated. It is said that, "Qi is the commander of the blood and blood is the mother of qi." This means that it is qi which moves the blood but that it is the blood which provides the nourishment and physical foundation for the creation and existence of the qi.

In Chinese medicine, blood provides the following functions for the body:

1. Nourishment

Blood nourishes the body. Along with qi, the blood goes to every part of the body. When the blood is insufficient, function decreases and tissue atrophies or shrinks.

2. Moistening

Blood moistens the body tissues. This includes the skin, eyes, and ligaments and tendons or what are simply called the sinews of the body in Chinese medicine. Thus blood insufficiency can cause drying out and consequent stiffening of various body tissues throughout the body.

3. Blood provides the material foundation for the spirit or mind.

In Chinese medicine, the mind and body are not two separate things. The spirit is nothing other than a great accumulation of qi. The blood (yin) supplies the material support and nourishment for the spirit (yang) so that it accumulates, becomes bright (*i.e.*, conscious and clever), and stays rooted in the body. If the blood becomes insufficient, the mind can "float," causing problems like insomnia, agitation, and unrest.

Essence

Along with qi and blood, essence is one of the three most important constituents of the body. Essence is the most fundamental, essential material the body utilizes for its growth, maturation, and reproduction. There are two forms of this essence. We inherit essence from our parents and we also produce our own essence from the food we eat, the liquids we drink, and the air we breathe.

The essence which comes from our parents is what determines our basic constitution, strength, and vitality. We each have a finite, limited amount of this inherited essence. It is important to protect and conserve this essence because all bodily functions depend upon it, and, when it is gone, we die. Thus the depletion of essence has serious implications for our overall health and well-being. Happily, the essence derived from food and drink helps to bolster and support this inherited essence. Thus, if we eat well and do not consume more qi and blood than we create each day, then when we sleep at night, this surplus qi and more especially blood is transformed into essence.

Spirit

Spirit in Chinese medicine means one's mental-emotional faculties. Basically, it is a way of saying consciousness. In Chinese medicine, this term does not have any religious or "spiritual" connotation. Spirit in a Chinese medical sense is nothing other than the accumulation of qi and blood in the heart. If enough qi and blood accumulates in the heart, then this gives rise to consciousness which in Chinese medicine is called the spirit. Because of the interrelationship between the essence, the qi, and the spirit, sometimes consciousness is called the "essence spirit." If one is particularly talking about the emotions, then the compound term "spirit will" (will meaning desire) is commonly used. At other times, because the spirit is associated with mental clarity, the compound term "spirit brightness" or "spirit brilliance" is used. In order for there to be spirit, there must be sufficient qi. But in order for that spirit to be calm and healthy, there must be sufficient blood to nourish the spirit and keep it under control. Because the spirit made from qi is inherently yang in nature, it tends to stir or become restless if yin blood does not nourish and "mother" it. Therefore, normal mental clarity is referred to as "having spirit", while emotional upsetment is referred to as "spirit not quiet" or "restless spirit."

On the one hand, the spirit is made up from the qi and blood which are produced by the viscera and bowels we will talk about next. On the other, the qi and, therefore, the spirit are affected by external stimuli. Thus, there is no dichotomy or division in Chinese medicine between the psychological and biological. The

14

mind arises as a function of the viscera and bowels, but the functioning of the viscera and bowels is affected by the experiences of the mind and emotions. In fact, every thought in the mind or felt emotion is nothing other than the experience of the movement of qi. If one changes the way the qi moves, one changes one's mental-emotional experience, while changing one's mind and emotions changes the way the qi moves. Hence the qi and the spirit or mind are not two different things but rather a single reality.

The Viscera & Bowels

In Chinese medicine, the internal organs (called viscera so as not to become confused with the Western biological entities of the same name) have a wider area of function and influence than in Western medicine. Each viscus has distinct responsibilities for maintaining the physical and psychological health of the individual. When thinking about the internal viscera according to Chinese medicine, it is more accurate to view them as spheres of influence or a network that spreads throughout the body, rather than as a distinct and separate physical organ as described by Western science. This is why the famous German sinologist, Manfred Porkert, refers to them as orbs rather than as organs. In Chinese medicine, the relationship between the various viscera and other parts of the body is made possible by the channel and network vessel system which we will discuss below.

In Chinese medicine, there are five main viscera which are relatively yin and six main bowels which are relatively yang. The five yin viscera are the heart, lungs, liver, spleen, and kidneys. The six yang bowels are the stomach, small intestine, large intestine, gallbladder, urinary bladder, and a system that Chinese medicine refers to as the triple burner. All the functions of the entire body are subsumed or described under these eleven organs or spheres of influence. Thus Chinese medicine *as a system* does not have a pancreas, a pituitary gland, or the

15

ovaries. Nonetheless, all the functions of these Western organs are described under the Chinese medical system of the five viscera and six bowels.

Within this system, the five viscera are the most important. These are the organs that Chinese medicine says are responsible for the creation and transformation of qi and blood and the storage of essence. For instance, the kidneys are responsible for the excretion of urine but are also responsible for hearing, the strength of the bones, sex, reproduction, maturation and growth, the lower and upper back, and the lower legs in general and the knees in particular.

Visceral Correspondences

Organ	Tissue	Sense	Emotion
Kidneys	bones/ head hair	hearing	fear
Liver	sinews	sight	anger
Spleen	flesh	taste	thinking/ worry
Lungs	skin/body hair	smell	grief/ sadness
Heart	blood vessels	speech	joy/fright

This points out that the Chinese viscera may have the same name and even some overlapping functions but yet are quite different from the organs of modern Western medicine. Each of the five Chinese medical viscera also has a corresponding tissue, sense, and emotion related to it. These are outlined in the table above.

In addition, each Chinese medical viscus or bowel possesses both a yin and a yang aspect. The yin aspect of a viscus or bowel refers to its substantial nature or tangible form. Further, an organ's yin is responsible for the nurturing, cooling, and moistening of that viscus or bowel. The yang aspect of the viscus or bowel represents its functional activities or what it does. An organ's yang aspect is also warming. These two aspects, yin and yang, form and function, cooling and heating, when balanced create good health. However, if either yin or yang becomes too strong or too weak, the result will be disease.

All five viscera are potentially associated with the causes and mechanisms of depression, while only two of the six bowels are —the gallbladder and stomach. Below are the main statements of fact in Chinese medicine regarding these five viscera and two bowels which we will be using in our description of the diagnosis and treatment of depression. For a more complete listing of the statements of fact pertaining to all the five viscera and six bowels, see Bob Flaws's *Statements of Fact in Traditional Chinese Medicine*.

The kidneys

In Chinese medicine, the kidneys are considered to be the foundation of our life. Because the developing fetus looks like a large kidney and because the kidneys are the main viscus for the storage of inherited essence, the kidneys are referred to as the prenatal root. Thus keeping the kidney qi strong and kidney yin and yang in relative balance is considered essential to good health and longevity. Some basic Chinese medical statements of fact about the kidneys which are relevant to the mechanisms of depression are:

1. The kidneys are considered responsible for human reproduction, development, and maturation.
These are the same functions we used when describing the essence. This is because the essence is stored in the kidneys. Health problems related to reproduction, development, and maturation are considered to be problems of the kidney essence.

Excessive sexual activity, drug use, or simple prolonged over-exhaustion can all damage and consume kidney essence. Kidney essence is also consumed by the simple act of aging.

2. The kidneys are the foundation of water metabolism.
The kidneys work in coordination with the lungs and spleen to insure that water is spread properly throughout the body and that excess water is excreted as urination. Therefore, problems such as edema, excessive dryness, or excessive day or nighttime urination can indicate a weakness of kidney function.

3. The kidneys store the will.
Will here means desire. If kidney qi is insufficient, this aspect of our human nature can be weakened. Conversely, pushing ourselves to extremes, such as long distance running or cycling, can eventually exhaust our kidneys.

4. Fear is the emotion associated with the kidneys.
This means that fear can manifest when the kidney qi is insufficient. Vice versa, constant or excessive fear can damage the kidneys and make them weak.

The liver

In Chinese medicine, the liver is associated with one's emotional state, with digestion, and with menstruation in women. The basic Chinese medical statements of facts concerning the liver include:

1. The liver controls coursing and discharge.
Coursing and discharge refer to the uninhibited spreading of qi to every part of the body. If the liver is not able to maintain the free and smooth flow of qi throughout the body, multiple physical and emotional symptoms can develop. This function of the liver is most easily damaged by emotional causes and, in particular, by anger and frustration. For example, if the liver is stressed due to pent-up anger, the flow of liver qi can become depressed or stagnate.

18

Liver qi stagnation can cause a wide range of health problems, including PMS, chronic digestive disturbance, depression, and insomnia. Therefore, it is essential to keep our liver qi flowing freely.

2. The liver stores the blood.
This means that the liver regulates the amount of blood in circulation. In particular, when the body is at rest, the blood in the extremities returns to the liver. As an extension of this, it is said in Chinese medicine that the liver is yin in form but yang in function. Thus the liver requires sufficient blood to keep it and its associated tissues moist and supple, cool and relaxed.

3. The emotion associated with the liver is anger.
Anger is the emotion that typically arises when the liver is diseased and especially when its qi does not flow freely. Conversely, anger damages the liver. Thus the emotions related to the stagnation of qi in the liver are frustration, anger, and rage.

The heart

Although the heart is the emperor of the body-mind according to Chinese medicine, it does not play as large a role in the creation and treatment of disease as one might think. Rather than the emperor initiating the cause of disease, in Chinese medicine, mostly enduring disease eventually affects the heart. Especially in terms of depression, disturbances of the heart tend to be secondary rather than primary. By this we mean that first some other viscus or bowel becomes diseased and then the heart feels the negative effect. The basic statements of fact about the heart in Chinese medicine which relate to depression are:

1. The heart governs the blood.
This means that it is the heart qi which "stirs" or moves the blood within its vessels. This is roughly analogous to the heart's pumping the blood in Western medicine. The pulsation of the

19

blood through the arteries due to the contraction of the heart is referred to as the "stirring of the pulse." In fact, the Chinese word for pulse and vessel is the same. So this could also be translated as the "stirring of the vessels."

2. The heart stores the spirit.

The spirit refers to the mind in Chinese medicine. Therefore, this statement underscores that mental function, mental clarity, and mental equilibrium are all associated with the heart. If the heart does not receive enough qi or blood or if the heart is disturbed by something, the spirit may become restless and this may produce symptoms of mental-emotional unrest, heart palpitations, insomnia, profuse dreams, etc.

3. The heart governs the vessels.

This statement is very close to number one above. The vessels refer to the blood vessels and also to the pulse.

4. The heart governs speech.

If heart function becomes abnormal, this may be reflected in various speech problems and especially in raving and delirious speech, muttering to oneself, and speaking incoherently.

5. The heart opens into the portal of the tongue.

Because the heart has a special relationship with the tip of the tongue, heart problems may manifest as sores on the tip of the tongue.

6. Joy is the emotion associated with the heart.

The word joy has been interpreted by both Chinese and Westerners in different ways. On the one hand, joy can mean over-excitation, in which case excessive joy can cause problems with the Chinese medical functions of the heart in terms of governing the blood and storing the spirit. On the other hand, joy may be seen as an antidote to the other six emotions of Chinese medicine. From this point of view, joy causes the flow of qi (and therefore blood) to relax and become more moderate and harmonious. If some other emotion causes the qi to become bound or move chaotically, then joy can make it relax and flow normally and smoothly.

The spleen

The spleen is less important in Western medicine than it is in Chinese medicine. Since at least the Yuan dynasty (1280-1368 CE), the spleen has been one of the two most important viscera of Chinese medicine (the other being the kidneys). In Chinese medicine, the spleen plays a pivotal role in the creation of qi and blood and in the circulation and transformation of body fluids. Therefore, when it comes to the spleen, it is especially important not to think of this Chinese viscus in the same way as the Western spleen. The main statements of fact concerning the spleen in Chinese medicine, which help explain depression are:

1. The spleen governs movement and transformation.
This refers to the movement and transformation of foods and liquids through the digestive system. In this case, movement and transformation may be paraphrased as digestion. However, secondarily, movement and transformation also refer to the movement and transformation of body fluids through the body. It is the spleen qi which is largely responsible for controlling liquid metabolism in the body.

2. The spleen restrains the blood.
As mentioned above, one of the five functions of the qi is to restrain the fluids of the body, including the blood, within their proper channels and reservoirs. If the spleen qi is healthy and abundant, then the blood is held within its vessels properly. However, if the spleen qi becomes weak and insufficient, then the blood may flow outside its channels and vessels resulting in various types of pathological bleeding. This includes various types of pathological bleeding associated with the menstrual cycle.

21

3. The spleen stores the constructive.

The constructive is one of the types of qi in the body. Specifically, it is the qi responsible for nourishing and constructing the body and its tissues. This constructive qi is closely associated with the process of digestion and the creation of qi and blood out of food and liquids. If the spleen fails to store or runs out of constructive qi, then the person becomes hungry on the one hand, and eventually becomes fatigued on the other.

4. Thought is the emotion associated with the spleen.

In the West, we do not usually think of thought as an emotion per se. Be that as it may, in Chinese medicine it is classified along with anger, joy, fear, grief, and melancholy. In particular, thinking, or perhaps I should say over-thinking, causes the spleen qi to bind. This means that the spleen qi does not flow harmoniously and this typically manifests as loss of appetite, abdominal bloating after meals, and indigestion.

5. The spleen is the source of engenderment and transformation.

Engenderment and transformation refer to the creation or production of the qi and blood out of the food and drink we take in each day. If the spleen receives adequate food and drink and then properly transforms that food and drink, it engenders or creates the qi and blood. Although the kidneys and lungs also participate in the creation of the qi, while the kidneys and heart also participate in the creation of the blood, the spleen is the pivotal viscus in both processes, and spleen qi weakness and insufficiency is a leading cause of qi and blood insufficiency and weakness.

The lungs

The lungs are not one of the main Chinese viscera in the cause of depression. However, like the heart, the lungs often bear the brunt of disease processes initiated in other viscera and bowels. As in Western medicine, the lungs are often subject to externally invading pathogens resulting in respiratory tract diseases.

However, the lungs sphere of influence also includes the skin and fluid metabolism. The main statements of fact regarding the lungs in Chinese medicine are:

1. The lungs govern the qi.
Specifically, the lungs govern the downward spread and circulation of the qi. It is the lung qi which moves all the rest of the qi in the body out to the edges and from the top of the body downward. Thus the lung qi is something like a sprinkler spraying out qi. As an extension of this, this downward qi then makes sure body fluids are moved throughout the body and eventually down to the kidneys and bladder and, eventually, out of the body.

2. The lungs govern the defensive exterior.
We said above that the qi defends the body against invasion by external pathogens. In Chinese medicine, the exterior most layer of the body is the area where the defensive qi circulates and the place where this defense, therefore, takes place. In particular, it is the lungs which govern this defensive qi. If the lungs function normally and there is sufficient defensive qi, then the body cannot be invaded by external pathogens. If the lungs are weak and the defensive qi is insufficient, then external pathogens may easily invade the exterior of the body, causing complaints such as colds, flus, and allergies.

The gallbladder

The main statements of fact concerning the gallbladder in terms of depression in Chinese medicine are:

1. The gallbladder governs decision.
In Chinese medicine, the liver is likened to a general who plans strategy for the body, while the gallbladder is likened to a judge. According to this point of view, if a person lacks gallbladder qi, they will have trouble making decisions. In addition, they will be timid. While courage in the West is associated with the heart

(*coeur* = courage), bravery in the East is associated with the gallbladder. Actually, this is also an old Western idea as well. When someone is very forward and brazen, we say that "They have gall." Conversely, if someone is excessively timid, this may be due to gallbladder qi vacuity or insufficiency. In Chinese medicine, this is called "gallbladder timidity." It is common to have people describe their experience of depression as an inability to make decisions, feeling insecure and having very low self-esteem.

2. The liver and gallbladder have the same palace.
This statement underscores the particularly close relationship between the liver and gallbladder.

3. The eleven viscera depend on the gallbladder.

4. If there is qi because of a robust gallbladder, evils are not able to enter.
These two statements about the gallbladder are very similar to statements in Chinese medicine about the heart which say that the heart is the sovereign of the body and that if spirit abides (in the heart), then evils cannot enter. Both these statements elevate the gallbladder to a place of importance in the body it does not hold in Western medicine and, in a way, link the gallbladder to the heart and its spirit.

The stomach

There are a number of important statements of fact concerning the stomach in Chinese medicine due to the stomach's pivotal role in digestion and, therefore, in the creation of qi and blood. Below we will only discuss those statements which we will use later in our discussion of the disease causes and disease mechanisms of depression in Chinese medicine.

1. The stomach governs intake.
This means that the stomach is the first to receive foods and drinks ingested into the body.

2. The stomach governs downbearing of the turbid.

The process of digestion in Chinese medicine is likened to the process of fermentation and then distillation. The stomach is the fermentation tun wherein foods and liquids are "rottened and ripened." This rottening and ripening allows for the separation of clear and turbid parts of the digestate. The spleen sends the clear parts upward to the lungs and heart to become the qi and blood respectively. The stomach's job is to send the turbid part down to be excreted as waste from the large intestine and bladder.

3. Stomach heat may exploit the heart.

If, for any reason, abnormal or pathological heat collects in the stomach, because heat is yang and has an innate tendency to move upward and outward, and because the heart is located above the stomach in Chinese medicine, heat in the stomach may exploit or harass the heart above.

4. The stomach is the origin of the defensive qi.

We have seen above that the defensive qi is the qi which defends the exterior of the body from invasion by external pathogens. This defensive qi's other job is to warm the internal organs. According to some points of view, the stomach is the origin of the defensive qi. This is because it is in the stomach that the clear and turbid parts of the digestate are separated, and the defensive qi is made out of a further refinement of the turbid part of this digestate.

Above we mentioned that there are five viscera and six bowels. The sixth bowel is called the triple burner. It is said in Chinese that, "The triple burner has a function but no form." The name triple burner refers to the three main areas of the torso. The upper burner is the chest. The middle burner is the space from the bottom of the ribcage to the level of the navel. The lower burner is the lower abdomen below the navel. These three spaces are called burners because all of the functions and trans-formations of the viscera and bowels which they contain are "warm" transformations similar to food cooking in a pot on a stove or similar to an alchemical transformation in a furnace. In fact, the triple burner is nothing other than a generalized concept of how the other viscera and bowels function together as an organic unit in terms of the digestion of foods and liquids and the circulation and transformation of body fluids.

As we will see below there are channels connected with each viscus and each bowel. There is a channel however, which is very important in the treatment of depression, which does not correspond to any viscera or bowel. This channel, the hand *jue yin* channel also known as the pericardium functions both as an extension of the heart in relation to the spirit and regulates the flow of qi mediated by the liver in the upper and middle burners.

The Channels & Network Vessels

Each viscus and bowel has a corresponding channel with which it is connected. In Chinese medicine, the inside of the body is made up of the viscera and bowels. The outside of the body is composed of the sinews and bones, muscles and flesh, and skin and hair. It is the channels and network vessels (*i.e.*, smaller connecting vessels) which connect the inside and the outside of the body. It is through these channels and network vessels that the viscera and bowels connect with their corresponding body tissues.

The channels and network vessel system is a unique feature of traditional Chinese medicine. These channels and vessels are different from the circulatory, nervous, or lymphatic systems. The earliest reference to these channels and vessels is in *Nei Jing (Inner Classic)*, a text written around the 2nd or 3rd century BCE.

The channels and vessels perform two basic functions. They are the pathways by which the qi and blood circulate through the body and between the organs and tissues. Additionally, as mentioned above, the channels connect the viscera and bowels internally with the

26

exterior part of the body. This channel and vessel system functions in the body much like the world information communication network. The channels allow the various parts of our body to cooperate and interact to maintain our lives.

This channel and network vessel system is complex. There are 12 primary channels, six yin and six yang, each with a specific pathway through the external body and connected with an internal organ (see diagram below). There are also extraordinary vessels, sinew channels, channel divergences, main network vessels, and ultimately countless finer and finer network vessels permeating the entire body. All of these form a closed loop or circuit similar to but distinct from the Western circulatory system.

Acupuncture points are places located on the major channels where there is a special concentration of qi and blood. Because of the relatively more qi and blood accumulated at these places, the sites act as switches which can potentially control the flow of qi and blood in the channel on which the point is located. By stimulating these points in any of a number of different ways, one can speed up or slow down, make more or reduce, warm or cool down the qi and blood flowing in the channels and vessels. The main ways of stimulating these points and thus adjusting the flow of qi and blood in the channels and vessels is to needle them and to heat them by moxibustion.[2] Other commonly used ways of stimulating these points and thus adjusting the qi and blood flowing through the channels and vessels are massage, cupping, the application of magnets, and the application of various herbal medicinals. If the channels and vessels are the pathways over which the qi and blood flow, then the acupuncture points are the places where this flow can be adjusted.

---

[2] Moxibustion refers to adding heat to an acupuncture point or area of the body by burning a dried herb, Folium Artemisae Argyii (*Ai Ye*), Oriental mugwort, on, over, or near the area to be warmed.

27

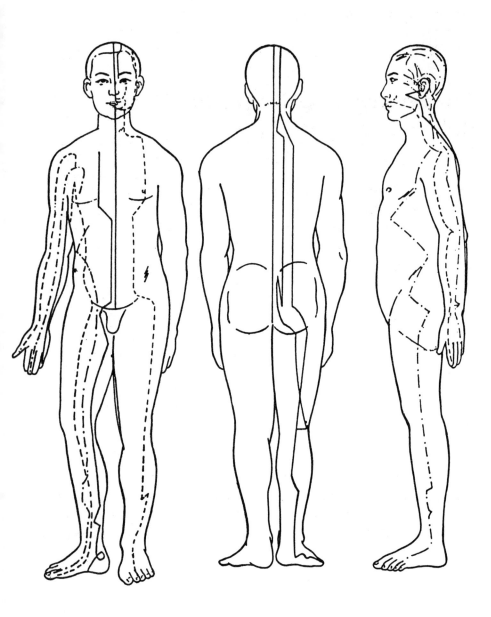

The Concept of Qi Stagnation & Its Relationship to the Liver

As we will soon see, the concept of qi stagnation is essential to understanding the Chinese mechanisms of depression. Therefore, this chapter is devoted to a discussion of the causation and ramifications of qi stagnation. In particular, we will also look at qi stagnation from the point of view of the female menstrual cycle and see how aging affects qi stagnation in both men and women.

As we saw above, the liver spreads the qi and maintains the smooth and unobstructed flow of qi. Because the qi moves the blood, this smooth and uninhibited flow of qi insures the free and easy flow of blood. It is said in Chinese medicine that, "The liver is the temperamental viscus" and that, "The liver likes to spread freely." This means that the liver is typically the first organ negatively affected by mental-emotional stress and is particularly susceptible to a thwarting of one's desires. If the function of the liver is negatively affected by frustration, suppressed emotion, or stress (which is basically desiring to do more than one can in a given situation), this means the liver's coursing and discharging is affected. In this case, the qi does not spread freely throughout the body, but rather becomes stagnant. Technically, this is referred to as liver depression qi stagnation, and its main cause is emotional stress and frustration.[3]

Accumulation & counterflow

If the liver becomes depressed and the qi consequently becomes stagnant, the qi will tend to back up and accumulate. After all, it has to go somewhere. This means that one of the first symptoms of qi stagnation is fullness and distention in the areas traversed by the channels and vessels connected to the liver. The liver channel traverses or connects with the insides of the legs and thighs, the pelvic region, the upper abdomen, the chest, the throat, gums, eyes, and top of the head. The liver channel is connected to the hand *jue yin* pericardium channel which is a kind of extension of the liver channel in the upper part of the body. This channel traverses the insides of the arms but especially the upper abdomen and the chest. The liver channel also connects with the gallbladder channel. The gallbladder channel is the yang paired channel to the yin liver channel. The course of the gallbladder channel runs up the outsides of the legs, through the pelvis, up the sides of the flanks, the sides of the neck, and the sides of the head. Because qi is yang, stagnant and, therefore, accumulated qi, which originates in a yin viscus and channel often moves into its paired yang channel. So the symptoms of liver depression qi stagnation often manifest as fullness, distention, and lack of free flow on the gallbladder channel. In addition, because the qi is yang, it has an innate tendency to move in the yang direction—upward. If the qi

---

[3] Throughout this book the word depression is used in two different but related ways. When occurring alone, the word depression primarily means the Western disease category of depression. When combined with the word liver, as in liver depression qi stagnation, it refers to a particular Chinese disease mechanism and pattern of disharmony. Although it is our thesis that the overwhelming majority of sufferers of the disease depression manifest, at least in part, the Chinese pattern of liver depression qi stagnation, there is no tit-for-tat identity between these two concepts. As we will see below, liver depression is only one contributing factor in most people's depression even if it is a pivotal one.

becomes stagnant and accumulates, it will eventually counterflow upward, although it may also counterflow horizontally as well.

Depressive heat

There is yet another consequence of the qi's being yang when it becomes depressed and stagnant. What happens to air which is pumped into a tire as the pressure in that tire begins to mount? It becomes hot. If enough qi becomes trapped and depressed, it will eventually transform into heat. This heat is technically called depressive heat in Chinese medicine. It is the result of extreme or long-term stagnation of the liver qi. Therefore, there are three main groups of symptoms associated with liver depression qi stagnation due to emotional stress and frustration: 1) fullness and distention, 2) counterflow (*i.e.*, the venting of excessive liver qi to an area of the body it should not), and 3) depressive or transformative heat. Because heat typically moves upward due to its inherently yang nature, this depressive heat may negatively affect the function of the organs and tissues located above the liver. These include the stomach, heart, and lungs in terms of viscera and bowels, and the head, mouth, nose, ears, and eyes in terms of body parts. Since the spirit resides in the heart, upwardly counterflowing depressive heat may disturb the heart spirit causing it to become restless.

Qi stagnation and the blood & body fluids

Because it is the qi which moves and transforms the blood and body fluids and, if the qi stops, so do these, long-term qi stagnation may result in blood stasis and damp accumulation. If dampness lingers and is not transformed, it may congeal into phlegm. This phlegm may then lodge in the viscera or bowels, the channels or network vessels, or in the body's various orifices, obstructing the flow of qi even more and, therefore, the function of those viscera, channels, or orifices. Similarly, blood stasis, dampness accumulation, or phlegm obstruction occurring due to any reason may cause or aggravate qi stagnation. Once these pathological yin substances exist in the body, they hinder and impede the free and easy flow of yang qi. Thus, qi stagnation may

31

give rise to blood stasis, dampness, or phlegm, while blood stasis, dampness, and phlegm may cause or aggravate qi stagnation.

The menstrual cycle in Chinese medicine

Because statistically more women suffer from depression than men,[4] we need to look at the Chinese theories which explain this fact. It is said in Chinese medicine that men and women are basically the same. However, women have a uterus and thus they menstruate, can conceive, give birth, and lactate. The fact that more women are diagnosed with depression is due to the mechanics of their menstrual cycle *vis à vis* liver depression qi stagnation.

The menses themselves are a discharge of blood. For this discharge to take place, two things have to occur. First, a superabundance of blood must accumulate in the uterus for it to eventually spill over as the menstruate. And secondly, the qi and blood must be freely and uninhibitedly flowing in order to allow this brimming over. This means that, in order to understand menstruation, one must understand how blood is created and what might affect the free and uninhibited flow of qi and blood.

The creation of blood

There are three viscera which participate in the creation of the blood. These are the kidneys, spleen, and heart. The heart is the place where the blood is "turned red" or finally created. However, first the spleen must send up the finest essence of food and liquids extracted in the process of digestion. If the spleen does not send up this finest essence of food and liquids there will be insufficient supplies for the heart to transform these into blood. In addition, the kidneys must send up some essence to also participate in the creation of blood. One can think of this as

---

[4] *The Merck Manual of Diagnosis and Therapy*, ed. by Robert Berkow, Merck, Sharp & Dohme Research Laboratories, Rahway, NJ, 1987, p. 1517

somewhat similar to adding some sourdough starter in order to make a new batch of sourdough bread.

In other words, if the kidneys lack sufficient essence, if the spleen fails to digest the finest essence of food and liquids and send this upward, and if the heart, for any reason, cannot fufill its function of "turning the blood red", then there may be insufficient creation of blood. In addition, it is the heart's job to spread the blood to the rest of the body and eventually move it down to the uterus. It is said in Chinese medicine that first the blood goes to nourish and moisten the viscera and bowels. Then it goes into the channels and vessels. From there it nourishes and moistens the rest of the tissues of the body, and what collects in the uterus is what is left over after the blood has performed all these other jobs. When enough blood collects in the uterus to fill it, it overflows as the menses. Typically, a young to middle-aged, healthy woman will produce such a superabundance accumulating in the uterus once every 28-30 days.

The control of the blood

Although normal menstruation cannot occur if there is insufficient blood accumulated in the uterus, it can occur either too early or too late if the flow of blood is not controlled properly. Just as there are three viscera which engender and transform the blood, there are three viscera which govern or control the blood. These are the heart, liver, and spleen. It is said that the heart qi governs the blood. Above we have seen that this means that it is the heart qi which "stirs" or pushes the blood. If the heart qi does not move the blood, the blood cannot move on its own. Thus it is said:

If the qi moves, the blood moves. If the qi stops, the blood stops.

In actual fact, the heart gets its qi primarily from the spleen. So a sufficiency of spleen qi is necessary for there to be enough heart qi to move the blood. In addition, the spleen qi restrains and contains the blood within its channels and vessels. If the spleen

33

qi is too weak, it may allow the blood to seep out prematurely or it may not cut off menstruation when it should. And finally, the liver stores the blood. It is the liver's job to regulate the amount of blood in circulation. It is the liver qi which performs this function. If the liver qi spreads freely, then the blood moves. If the liver qi becomes depressed and stagnant, then the blood will also eventually become depressed and static.

One may find it hard at first to distinguish the difference between the spleen and the liver's role in maintaining the free and uninhibited flow of blood. It is the spleen qi ultimately (via the heart) which provides the motivating force behind the propulsion of the blood. It is the liver which allows the blood to flow freely through its channels and vessels. If, for instance, one has gas in their car and the car is in good working order, one may have the power to move one's car. However, if one is stopped at a red light, one may not have the permission to move the car even though the power is there. In terms of the heart, spleen and liver, the flow of blood is the same. The heart and spleen provide the motivating power, but it is the liver qi which allows that blood to flow freely or not.

If, for any reason, one of these three viscera does not function correctly in terms of the flow of blood, this may impede the free and timely flow of the menstruate. Conversely, the menstrual cycle places certain burdens on and affects these viscera in ways not experienced by men. The functions of the liver, heart, spleen, and kidneys may all be negatively impacted by the menstrual cycle and, as we will see below, these are the main viscera involved in depression.

The four phases of the menstrual cycle
Chinese gynecologists divide the menstrual cycle into four, roughly seven day periods. Phase one begins the day the menses end. If one counts the days of the menstrual cycle from the first day of the onset of menstruation, this means that phase one typically begins on day four, five, six, or seven. The uterus had

34

discharged its accumulated blood and this leaves the body relatively empty or vacuous of blood. Because blood is created, at least in part out of kidney essence and because, compared to yang qi, essence is a type of yin substance, during phase one, the body busies itself with making more yin and blood to replenish that which was discharged. Therefore, in Chinese gynecology, we say that phase one corresponds to yin and the emphasis in the body is on replenishing yin blood.

If the body is having a hard time replacing this blood due to kidney yin vacuity, the heart spirit may not receive enough blood to nourish it and thus it may become more restless than usual during this phase. Since yin controls yang, yang heat may flare upward to harass the spirit in the heart and the spirit may also become restless for this reason as well.

Phase two corresponds to the days surrounding ovulation. Up till now, the body has been replenishing its yin. However, for ovulation to occur, yin must transform into yang. This transformation of yin into yang corresponds to the rise in basal body temperature which occurs after ovulation.[5] If there is insufficient yin, it cannot transform into yang. Conversely, if there is insufficient yang, it cannot transform yin. In addition, if either the qi and blood are not flowing freely, this transformation may also be impeded. Generally, phase two corresponds to days 10-16 in the monthly cycle and it corresponds to yang in the same way that phase one corresponds to yin.

If yin has grown successfully during phase one, the growth of yang may begin to take off during phase two. Since yang is associated with heat, this means that yang heat may flare

---

[5] Basal body temperature refers to one's resting temperature when taken the first thing upon waking in the morning before getting up, dressing, eating, or doing anything else. It is analogous to one's resting pulse or one's basal metabolic rate. Plotting one's basal body temperature on a graph is one way of determining if and when a woman is ovulating.

upward disturbing the heart spirit and causing restlessness and agitation. In this case, heat added to liver depression may cause otherwise simple qi stagnation to turn into depressive heat or even fire. What was irritability may thus become irascibility, while feelings of fullness, distention, and oppression may all become aggravated by a vexatious feeling of heat and agitation or restlessness.

Phase three corresponds to the premenstruum and to the qi. For things to go as they should in the woman's body, yang qi must stay strong enough long enough and the qi must flow freely and in the right direction. Many of the signs and symptoms of premenstrual syndrome or PMS, including premenstrual depression or a worsening of chronic depression during this time every month, have to do with the yang qi not being strong enough *or* the qi (and therefore the blood) not flowing freely.

The yang qi is produced by the spleen and kidneys. If, for any reason, such as improper diet, excessive work, insufficient exercise, enduring disease, too much thinking and anxiety (spleen) or too much fear (kidneys), or simply aging, the spleen and/or kidneys become weak, symptoms such as fatigue, lack of will, listlessness, and somnolence may occur or worsen during the premenstruum when extra strains are placed on the functions of these two viscera.

In addition, because the liver's function of coursing and discharge is dependent on nourishment of the liver by the blood, if a woman has too little blood, when what blood she does have accumulates in the uterus prior to menstruation, this may leave the rest of her body "high and dry." That means liver function may be compromised, thus causing or worsening liver depression qi stagnation. It also means that the heart spirit may not receive its proper nourishment from the blood, thus causing it to become unquiet or restless. Therefore, there are a number of reasons why a woman might become more depressed and/or agitated during phase three of her menstrual cycle. Phase three is usually

36

counted from day 17 to the day before menstruation. However, in real life, phase three begins whenever a woman begins to feel the onset of cyclically recurring PMS.

Phase four is the menstruation itself. Since the onset of menstruation is counted as day one in the cycle, phase four may last anywhere from one or two days to six or seven depending on the individual woman's constitution and age. Because menstruation is a downward discharge of blood according to Chinese medicine, phase four corresponds to the blood. Typically, this discharge of blood and the qi that follows along with it is experienced as a reduction in any signs and symptoms associated with liver depression qi stagnation or depressive heat.

When looked at from this perspective, the menstrual cycle is made up of four (not always equal) segments corresponding to yin, yang, qi and blood. This relationship is shown in the chart below.

Qi, Blood, Yin & Yang vis-a-vis Menstrual Cycle

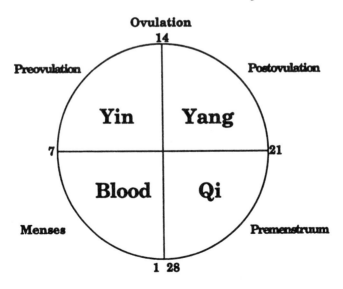

37

Health problems in women may occur in any of these four phases and may occur for reasons other than the dominant correspondence in that phase. However, when a problem occurs in a woman in any of these four phases, the Chinese doctor will first investigate to see if the dominant correspondence, whether yin, yang, qi, or blood, is behaving as it should at that time.

Aging and depression

In Chinese medicine, aging is seen as a decline in the production and free flow of the qi and blood in both men and women. Typically, first the spleen becomes weak, for instance at around 35 years of age in most women, and then, later on, due to the interdependence of the spleen and kidneys, the kidneys become vacuous and weak. Because both the spleen and kidneys work hand in hand in the production of the qi and blood, this production becomes scantier and scantier. Because the qi can only keep moving if there is sufficient qi being manufactured to keep propelling it, this decline in qi production is often accompanied by an inverse rise in signs and symptoms of liver depression and qi stagnation. This is aggravated by the decline in blood production, since blood is necessary to nourish and maintain the liver's coursing and discharge function. In addition, liver function is based on the yang warmth supplied to the liver by the kidneys. Hence decline and debility of kidney yang, what is also called the lifegate fire, adds to this aggravation of liver depression qi stagnation. Therefore, signs and symptoms associated with liver depression on the one hand and spleen-kidney vacuity on the other all tend to increase past a certain age. Since the heart spirit is nothing other than an accumulation of qi nourished and kept healthy by the blood, as qi production falls off, the spirit becomes weaker, *i.e.*, less clear or bright. As blood production falls off, the spirit becomes unquiet or restless. Hence, it is easy to see how a rise in the incidence or aggravation of existing depression in women is accounted for by Chinese medical theory.

Menopause and Chinese medicine

In women, eventually, the body in its wisdom recognizes it is not healthy to try to create qi and blood to nourish and empower the rest of the body at the same time as continuing to menstruate regularly with the loss of blood that that necessarily entails. Therefore, the body initiates a transformation which, from the Chinese medical point of view, is literally a "change in life." The Chinese medical literature does not say exactly how, but at some point, the heart ceases sending blood down to collect in the uterus. Just as maturation does not happen all at once, this process is also a gradual one in most women. Therefore, the menses do not just suddenly cease, but menopause is commonly preceded by months or even years of a certain amount of menstrual irregularity. Nevertheless, sooner or later, the heart stops sending blood down to the uterus. Instead, the kidneys are now free to send essence up to accumulate in the heart where it joins with the qi and blood sent up by the spleen and becomes spirit.

Thus the woman goes from mother of babies to mother of her tribe, the *sage femme* or wise woman full of spirit. If this change occurs smoothly, it naturally puts an end to any premenstual or menopausal depression. There is now more blood available to keep the liver harmonized and functioning correctly and there is more blood to nourish and quiet or calm the heart spirit. Because the spleen and kidneys do not have to create so much blood, they also do not have to expend so much qi in thier function. Hence they can spend more of the qi on propelling the qi through the body and warming the body, including the liver. All this results in the availability of more yang qi and less qi stagnation.

Unfortunately, the smooth cessation of menstruation is, like all other transformations in the body, dependent on the free flow of liver qi. Since there is no PMS without liver depression qi stagnation, women's menopausal complaints tend to be, both in Chinese theory and my own clinical experience (BF), proportional to the severity of their PMS. In other words, premenstrual and menopausal depression are ultimately not two separate diseases but an unfortunate continuum whose core issue is liver depression qi stagnation. Women with menopausal depression are hung up in the change. The change in the flow of qi and blood is not complete. Therefore, the above-described factors that normally make for a more relaxed liver and a calmer, more vigorous heart spirit after menopause do not occur. For more information about Chinese medicine and menopause, interested readers should see Honora Lee Wolfe's *Managing Menopause Naturally with Chinese Medicine* also published by Blue Poppy Press.

We have discussed a good bit of fairly complex Chinese medical theory above in this chapter and the one before it. You may not have gotten the technical implications of every point. However, at the least, you should have seen that Chinese medicine is based on a very elaborate, sophisticated, and, in its own way, logical theory. It is not a primitive folk medicine. The more of the above theory you can understand, the more the self-care and preventive techniques we suggest in the following pages will make sense. So please don't be dismayed if you have to read some of the above sentences twice.

The Chinese Medical Mechanisms of Depression

Chinese medicine has a very definite description of the causes and mechanisms of depression. The following description of these mechanisms is from *Zhong Yi Nei Ke Xue [The Study of Chinese Medicine Internal Medicine]* by Zhang Bo-ying *et al.* published in Shanghai in 1990. This is the basic textbook on internal medicine used at the Shanghai College of TCM and other Chinese provincial TCM colleges. All the other Chinese medical textbooks we have checked with basically agree with this description. It is a pretty standard one.

The disease causes & mechanisms of depression

The onset of depression is due to damage by the emotions. In particular, this means lack of fulfillment of one's desires. The liver qi thus becomes depressed and bound and gradually this leads to disharmony of the qi mechanism of the five viscera. This mainly affects the three viscera of the liver, spleen, and heart, causing loss of regulation of the qi and blood. This basic mechanism of liver depression qi stagnation then puts into motion other disease mechanisms which can be divided into two basic groups: 1) replete conditions where there is an excess of something which is pathological in the body, and 2) vacuity conditions where there is an insufficiency of something in the body necessary for healthy physiology or functioning.

1. Repletion disease mechanisms

If, due to depression and anger, there is loss of smooth flow of the qi, the liver loses its orderly reaching and the qi loses its coursing and discharging. If qi depression endures for many days, it may transform into fire. Qi stagnation may also lead to blood stasis. This means that the blood does not move freely but gathers and accumulates like silt in a river. If liver depression "reaches", *i.e.*, affects, the spleen, if thinking and worry are unresolved, or if overwork and fatigue damage the spleen, all these may make the spleen lose its fortification and movement. Because the spleen is in charge of the movement and transformation of body fluids, lack of spleen fortification and movement may lead to dampness brewing and engendering phlegm.[6] This then leads to qi stagnation and phlegm depression. Because the qi moves and transforms the foods and liquids taken into the stomach, if the qi becomes depressed and does not move, this may give rise to food stagnation. And further, because qi's nature is inherently warm, if qi becomes depressed and accumulates it may transform into depressive heat or fire.

2. Vacuity disease mechanisms

If the emotions are not fulfilled or satisfied, then liver depression may repress the spleen. Because the spleen is the source of qi and blood engenderment and transformation, this may result in consumption and damage of the heart qi. The constructive and blood are progressively consumed and the heart loses its nourishment, while the spirit loses its treasuring or storage. This is called anxiety and depression damaging the spirit and can lead to disquietude of the heart spirit. If such depression damaging the spleen goes on for a long time with decreased and scanty

---

[6] In Chinese medicine, phlegm is nothing other than congealed dampness. Dampness may be congealed into phlegm for any of three reasons. A) If dampness gathers and collects and is not moved and transformed for a long time, it may congeal into phlegm. B) If heat stews the juices, it may cook or brew the body fluids into phlegm. And C) cold may freeze or congeal dampness into phlegm.

eating and drinking, then the qi and blood may become insufficient due to lack of a source for their engenderment and transformation. In that case, the heart and spleen both become vacuous. If spleen vacuity endures, it may affect the kidneys, giving rise to kidney-spleen dual vacuity. As we have seen above, if depression endures, it may also transform into fire which easily damages and consumes yin blood. This then affects the kidneys, causing yin vacuity with fire effulgence.

Therefore, according to Chinese medical theory, depression is due to the emotions not flowing smoothly. The qi mechanism becomes depressed and stagnant and thus leads to the arisal of this disease. If it endures for many days or if it occurs in someone who is already depleted and weak, for instance due to enduring disease, old age, or the menstrual cycle, it can consume and damage the heart qi which is the basis of the spirit. If it goes on longer, it damages and consumes heart blood and spleen qi. If it goes on yet longer, it may also damage kidney yang and/or consume kidney yin. This means that depression of recent onset in relatively young people or those with robust constitutions primarily has to do with liver depression, depressive heat, and phlegm fire, while chronic depression or depression in those who are constitutionally weak, is a combination of liver depression with vacuity or insufficiencies of heart qi, spleen qi, heart blood, kidney yin and/or kidney yang. Because yin controls yang, if yin becomes insufficient to control yang, this gives rise to vacuity heat which rises upward in the body to disturb the spirit in the heart.

In addition, the above disease mechanisms may be aggravated or ameliorated by a number of other factors besides emotional stress and frustration. While lack of free flow of the emotions may be the primary cause of depression, diet and exercise also play very important roles. For instance, if one eats or drinks a lot of fried, fatty, greasy, spicey, peppery, "hot" foods, this makes it all the more likely that simple liver depression will transform into depressive heat. If one eats a lot of fatty, greasy foods or eats a lot of dairy products and meat, these damp, phlegmatic foods make the formation of phlegm all the more likely. Eating too much sugar and sweets, including fruit juices, or eating a lot of chilled, frozen, or uncooked foods, all damage the spleen and tend to cause or aggravate dampness. Likewise, the spleen is damaged by too little exercise, too much work, and/or standing too long. While a good amount of exercise strengthens the spleen, moves the qi, and helps course a depressed, stagnant liver. Thus what one eats and how one lives one's life all play a part in either the production or prevention of depression according to Chinese medicine.

Further, because of various interrelationships between the five viscera and six bowels and the qi, blood, and body fluids, the basic disease mechanisms of depression described above may also cause other secondary pathological changes. For instance, under repletion disease mechanisms above, it is mentioned that qi stagnation may give rise to blood stasis. This is because the qi moves the blood, if the qi moves the blood moves, and if the qi stops, the blood stops. Therefore, it is not uncommon to find signs and symptoms of blood stasis in persons with enduring liver depression qi stagnation (and especially in women) even though blood stasis per se is not described in the Chinese medical literature as a cause of depression. Likewise, since the qi moves and transforms the digestate, if there is qi stagnation, it is easy for there also to be food stagnation. However, food stagnation is not listed as a direct disease mechanism of depression.

Based on our clinical experience applying this theory to Western patients with depression, liver depression qi stagnation due to emotional stress and frustration may cause depression all by itself. However, this is usually only the case in very acute and uncomplicated depressive episodes. In most cases, liver depression qi stagnation combines with and aggravates pre-existing tendencies to imbalances in other viscera and bowels. The specific mechanisms triggered by a failure in the functions of coursing and discharge determine the individual's symptoms of depression, the nature and duration of the depressive episode, and the prognosis and outcome of the treatment. Most major depressive episodes involve liver depression qi stagnation as a main component. In dysthymia as well as recurrent, chronic, and recalcitrant cases of depression, liver depression qi stagnation progresses further to affect the blood and body fluids or occurs on a background of long-standing constitutional insufficiency.

As the reader can see, in Chinese medicine, there are different causes and mechanisms for depression in different people. Some of the causes have to do with mental-emotional causes and reactions. Some have to do with either too much or too little exercise and activity. Some may be due to other diseases in the body. Some are related to age and body type. Yet others may be due to faulty diet. Since different people's depression has different underlying causes and disease mechanisms, no one treatment will be effective for everyone. More importantly, if one can identify their pattern of depression, one can immediately know what they as individuals should and should not do, eat or not eat. In that case, because just the right treatment is given to the right individual, there is healing without side effects or doctor-caused complications.

The Chinese Medical Treatment of Depression

The hallmark of professional Chinese medicine is what is known as "treatment based on pattern discrimination." Modern Western medicine bases its treatment on a disease diagnosis. This means that two patients diagnosed as suffering from the same disease will get the same treatment. Traditional Chinese medicine also takes the patient's disease diagnosis into account. However, the choice of treatment is not based on the disease so much as it is on what is called the patient's pattern, and it is treatment based on pattern discrimination which is what makes Chinese medicine the holistic, safe, and effective medicine it is.

In order to explain the difference between a disease and pattern, let us take headache for example. Everyone who is diagnosed as suffering from a headache has to, by definition, have some pain in their head. In modern Western medicine and other medical systems which primarily prescribe on the basis of a disease diagnosis, one can talk about "headache medicines." However, amongst headache sufferers, one may be a man and the other a woman. One may be old and the other young. One may be fat and the other skinny. One may have pain on the right side of her head and the other may have pain on the left. In one case, the pain may be throbbing and continuous, while the other person's pain may be very sharp but intermittent. In one case, they may also have indigestion, a tendency to loose stools, lack of warmth in their feet, red eyes, a dry mouth and desire for cold drinks, while the other person has a wet, weeping, crusty skin rash with

47

red borders, a tendency to hay fever, ringing in their ears, and dizziness when they stand up. In Chinese medicine just as in modern Western medicine, both these patients suffer from headache. That is their disease diagnosis. However, they also suffer from a whole host of other complaints, have very different types of headaches, and very different constitutions, ages, and sex. In Chinese medicine, the patient's pattern is made up from all these other signs and symptoms and other information. Thus, in Chinese medicine, the pattern describes *the totality of the person as a unique individual*. And in Chinese medicine, treatment is designed to rebalance that entire pattern of imbalance as well as address the major complaint or disease. Thus, there is a saying in Chinese medicine:

> One disease, different treatments
> Different diseases, same treatment

This means that, in Chinese medicine, two patients with the same named disease diagnosis may receive different treatments *if their Chinese medical patterns are different*, while two patients diagnosed with different named diseases may receive the same treatment *if their Chinese medical pattern is the same*. In other words, in Chinese medicine, treatment is predicated primarily on one's pattern discrimination, not on one's named disease diagnosis. Therefore, each person is treated individually.

Since every patient gets just the treatment which is right to restore balance to their particular body, there are also no unwanted side effects. Side effects come from forcing one part of the body to behave while causing an imbalance in some other part. The medicine may have fit part of the problem but not the entirety of the patient as an individual. This is like robbing Peter to pay Paul. Since Chinese medicine sees the entire body (and mind!) as a single, unified whole, curing imbalance in one area of the body while causing it in another is unacceptable.

Below is a description of the major Chinese medical patterns seen in patients with the modern Western disease of depression. They are a combination of patterns taken from *Zhong Yi Nei Ke Xue (The Study of Chinese Medicine Internal Medicine)* by Zhang Bo-ying *et al.* and *Xian Dai Nan Zhi Bing Zhong Yi Zhen Liao Xue (A Study of the Chinese Medical Diagnosis & Treatment of Modern, Difficult to Treat Diseases)* by Wu Jun-yu and Bai Yong -bo. Basically, these are the signs and symptoms associated with the disease mechanisms discussed in the previous chapter. Following these signs and symptoms are the treatment principles necessary to redress or correct the imbalance implied in the name of the pattern. These treatment principles tell a person what to do to correct each pattern. Anything which embodies or conforms to those principles will help the patient under discussion, while anything which goes against these principles will aggravate the person's condition.

Treatment based on pattern discrimination

Repletion patterns

Liver depression qi stagnation

Main symptoms: Irritability, a tendency to sigh, premenstrual breast distention and pain, chest oppression and rib-side pain, lower abdominal distention and pain, discomfort in the stomach and epigastrium, diminished appetite, possible delayed menstruation whose amount is either scanty or profuse, darkish, stagnant menstrual blood, the menses unable to come easily, a normal or slightly dark tongue with thin, slimy, white fur, and a bowstring,[7] fine pulse. In addition, when there is depression, there is also typically a desire *not* to see people and *not* to talk.

---

[7] There are 28 main pulse types in Chinese medicine, the bowstring pulse being one of these. It feels like its name implies—like a taut violin or bowstring. It is almost universally felt in women with PMS.

Analysis of symptoms: If the emotions damage the liver, it loses its orderly reaching. Therefore, there is emotional repression and depression and the emotions are not calm or quiet. The liver channel traverses the lower abdomen and mixes with the stomach. Then it spreads across the chest and sides of the ribs. Therefore, if there is liver qi depression and stagnation with lack of smooth flow of the qi mechanism, the qi becomes stagnant and the blood static. The liver network vessels lose their harmony, and therefore, one sees abdominal distention, chest oppression, rib-side pain, and even non-movement of menstruation in women. If the liver qi attacks the stomach, the stomach loses its harmony and downbearing. Therefore, there is epigastric oppression and belching and burping, lack of appetite, and, in some cases, even nausea and vomiting. If the liver assails the spleen, this leads to abdominal distention and loss of normalcy in defecation. The thin, slimy tongue fur and the bowstring pulse are signs of liver-stomach disharmony.

Treatment principles: Course the liver, rectify the qi, and resolve depression

Liver depression transforms heat

Main symptoms: All the above signs and symptoms plus the following differences. First, the patient is not just irritable, they are downright angry. Secondly, there is a bitter taste in their mouth in the mornings when they wake. And third, there is a red tongue with yellow fur and a bowstring, rapid pulse. Other symptoms may include tinnitus, headache, red eyes, dry mouth, dry, bound, constipated stools, violent outbursts of anger, cursing, shouting, and physically throwing or destroying things.

Analysis of symptoms: If qi depression transforms into fire, fire's nature is to flare upward. Therefore, it follows the liver vessels and moves upward. This results in headache, red eyes, and tinnitus. If liver fire attacks the stomach, the stomach and intestines will have heat. Therefore, the mouth is dry and there is a bitter taste, while the stools are constipated and bound. The emotional tension, agitation, and easy anger, the red tongue with yellow fur, and the bowstring, rapid pulse are all signs of liver fire.

Treatment principles: Course the liver and rectify the qi, clear heat and resolve depression

Liver blood stasis & stagnation

Main symptoms: Emotional depression, heart vexation and agitation, thoughts of suicide, a dark, dusky facial complexion, rib-side and flank distention and pain, possible amenorrhea or painful menstruation in women, a dark, purplish tongue, possibly having static spots or macules, white fur, and a deep, bowstring, or choppy pulse

Analysis of symptoms: If liver depression endures or is very bad, the qi may fail to move the blood. The blood, therefore, becomes static due to the qi's being stagnant. Thus, there are a combination of liver depression qi stagnation signs and symptoms, such as the rib-side distention and bowstring pulse along with blood stasis symptoms, such as lower abdominal or menstrual pain, a purple tongue, or a choppy pulse.

Treatment principles: Course the liver and move the qi, quicken the blood and transform stasis

Phlegm dampness obstruction and stagnation

Main symptoms: Discomfort within the throat as if there were something obstructing and blocking the throat which can neither be swallowed down or spit out, oppression within the chest, possible simultaneous rib-side pain, slimy, white tongue fur, and a bowstring, slippery pulse

Analysis of symptoms: If liver depression assails the spleen and the spleen movement loses its fortification, then dampness will be engendered and this may gather into phlegm. Phlegm and qi thus become depressed and bound in the chest and above the diaphragm. Therefore, one sees discomfort within the throat as if there were something blocking and obstructing it which can neither be swallowed down nor spit out. This is called plum pit qi because the Chinese liken this sensation to having a plum pit stuck in your throat. If qi loses its soothing, then there is oppression within the chest. The rib-sides are the place where the liver channel spreads across. If the channels and network vessels of the liver become depressed and stagnant, then there is rib-side pain. The slimy, white tongue fur and the bowstring, slippery pulse are symptoms of liver depression mixed with phlegm dampness.

Treatment principles: Transform phlegm, disinhibit the qi, and resolve depression

Phlegm fire harassing the spirit

Main symptoms: Insomnia, a heavy, full, stuffy, or tight feeling in the head, excessive or profuse phlegm, chest oppression,[8] aversion to food, burping and belching, acid regurgitation, possible nausea, heart vexation,[9] a bitter taste in the mouth, vertigo and dizziness, slimy, yellow tongue fur, and a slippery, rapid, possibly also bowstring pulse. In cases of depression, the person will feel both profoundly apathetic and tired yet restless and anxious or may alternate between one and the other.

---

[8] Chest oppression refers to a feeling of tightness and stuffiness in the chest. As a reaction to this feeling, the person will often sigh in an attempt to inhale fresh air and exhale the pent-up stale air.

[9] Heart vexation refers to an irritating, possibly dry, hot sensation in the chest in front of the heart.

Analysis of symptoms: Basically, this pattern is the same as the one above it except for the addition of heat or fire. The manifestations of this heat are the heart vexation, agitation, and insomnia, the bitter taste in the mouth, the yellow tongue fur, and the rapid pulse.

Treatment principles: Transform phlegm and clear heat, harmonize the stomach and quiet the spirit.

Vacuity patterns

Anxiety & worry harassing the heart spirit

Main symptoms: Mental-emotional abstraction, restlessness, sorrow and anxiety, a tendency to crying, frequent yawning, a pale tongue with thin, white fur, and a bowstring, fine pulse

Analysis of symptoms: If anxiety and depression are not resolved, the heart qi is consumed and damaged and the qi and blood become depleted and unable to nourish the heart spirit. Therefore, one sees mental-emotional abstraction, restlessness, and other such symptoms. The pale tongue with thin, white fur and the bowstring, fine pulse are signs of qi depression and blood vacuity.

Treatment principles: Nourish the heart and quiet the spirit

Heart-spleen dual vacuity

Main symptoms: Excessive thinking with a tendency to worry, heart palpitations, gallbladder timidity, scanty sleep, poor memory , a lusterless facial complexion, dizziness, lassitude of the spirit, devitalized eating and drinking, a pale tongue, and a fine, weak pulse. In depressed patients exhibiting this pattern, there is pronounced confusion, lack of concentration, lack of strength in the arms and legs, and severe fatigue.

Analysis of symptoms: If the heart is taxed by thinking and worry, the heart and spleen may both become vacuous. The heart thus loses its nourishment and, therefore one sees heart palpitations, timidity, scanty sleep, and poor memory. The spleen and stomach are the source of the engenderment and transformation of the qi and blood. If the spleen does not fortify and move, then eating and drinking are diminished and scanty and the source of qi and blood is insufficient. Therefore, one sees a lusterless facial complexion, dizziness, lassitude of the spirit, fatigue, lack of strength, a pale tongue, and a fine, weak pulse.

Treatment principles: Fortify the spleen and nourish the heart, boost the qi and supplement the blood

Spleen-kidney yang vacuity

Main symptoms: Emotional listlessness and depression, a predilection to lie down with little stirring, heart vexation, fright and fear, heart palpitations and loss of sleep, a somber white facial complexion, impotence in men or involuntary seminal emission, clear, watery vaginal discharge in women, decreased or absent libido in both men and women, low back soreness, cold feet, a fat, pale tongue with possible teeth marks on its edges and white fur, and a deep, fine pulse

Analysis of symptoms: If spleen qi vacuity endures or worsens and reaches the kidneys, kidney yang may also become vacuous and insufficient. Therefore, the signs and symptoms of qi vacuity are even more pronounced, such as a predilection to lie down and not move, plus there are symptoms of specifically kidney yang vacuity, such as lack of libido, low back soreness, and cold feet. Many women exhibit this pattern as they enter their perimenopausal years.

Treatment principles: Warm the kidneys and fortify the spleen, invigorate yang and boost the qi

54

Yin vacuity with fire effulgence

Main symptoms: Vertigo and dizziness, heart palpitations, scanty sleep, heart vexation, easy anger, possible involuntary seminal emission in men, low back soreness, menstrual irregularities in women, a red tongue, and a bowstring, fine, and rapid pulse. In patient's with depression, there is lots of anxiety, vexation and agitation, and restlessness.

Analysis of symptoms: If kidney yin is insufficient and the blood and body fluids are consumed by heat, depleted yin may not be able to control yang and hence yang floats upward. Therefore, one may see vertigo, dizziness, and easy anger. If there is yin and blood depletion and consumption, then the heart spirit loses its nourishment. In addition, yin vacuity gives rise to heat, and vacuity heat harasses the spirit. Therefore, there are heart palpitations, scanty sleep, and vexation and agitation. If kidney yin is insufficient, then the low back mansion loses its nourishment and thus there is low back soreness. Because there is yin vacuity with fire effulgence, effulgent fire harasses and stirs the essence chamber. Hence the essence is not secured and there is seminal emission. If the liver and kidneys lose their nourishment, the *chong* and *ren,* two vessels which in Chinese medicine are believed to control menstruation and which are related to the liver and kidneys respectively, will be unregulated. Therefore, there are menstrual irregularities. The red tongue and bowstring, fine, rapid pulse are both signs of yin vacuity.

Treatment principles: Enrich yin and clear heat, settle the heart and quiet the spirit

The real deal

Although textbook discriminations such as the one above make it seem like all the practitioner has to do is match up their patient's symptoms with one of the afore-mentioned patterns and

55

then prescribe the recommended guiding formula, in actual clinical practice, one usually encounters combinations of the above discreet patterns and their related disease mechanisms or progressions. For instance, liver depression transforming heat may be complicated by spleen qi and heart blood vacuity or by spleen qi and kidney yang vacuity. This, in turn may also be complicated by phlegm or blood stasis. Likewise, yin vacuity with fire effulgence may be complicated by liver depression and spleen qi vacuity, liver depression and blood stasis, or liver depression and phlegm.

In particular, liver depression and spleen vacuity go hand in hand in clinical practice. Rarely do you see one without the other, and especially in Westerners. Therefore, attention to and remedy of the causes and mechanisms of liver depression qi stagnation and spleen qi vacuity are almost always useful when dealing with depression. The *Nei Jing* or *Inner Classic*, the "bible" of Chinese medicine says, "If the liver is diseased, first treat the spleen." Once you have these two pivotal patterns, then all the rest of the patterns described above may easily evolve. In chronic, recurrent depression and dysthymia, usually there is long-standing phlegm obstruction, blood stasis, extreme insufficiency of qi and blood, or a combination of these elements. In bipolar disorder or manic-depression, there is always some sort of heat causing the mania. For instance, the three patterns Wu and Bai give for the manic part of bipolar disorder are 1) liver fire internally harassing, 2) liver-gallbladder depressive heat, and 3) exuberant heat damaging yin.

How This System Works in Real-life

Using all the above information on the theory of Chinese medicine and the patterns and their mechanisms of depression let's see how a Chinese doctor makes this system work in real-life.

Take Joan, for example, who we introduced at the beginning of this book. She has experienced depression on and off since she was about 13. In this most recent episode, she has been feeling depressed for a couple of months. She feels increasingly irritable and frustrated. She can't control her feelings, cries frequently, and wants only to be alone, feeling unmotivated and tired all the time. She wants to sleep constantly but has trouble falling asleep. Once she does fall asleep, her sleep is disturbed by intense dreams. Joan is 24 years old. She is slightly overweight, looks a bit puffy, but her musculature feels strong. She has trouble losing weight, eats constantly to calm herself down, and says she has gained a lot of weight lately. She feels bloated, burps a lot, and craves sweets. When she eats dairy, eggs, sugar, or fatty foods, her fatigue increases and she produces more mucous. Joan also says she feels worried, has trouble focusing, and feels overwhelmed by details. She is anxious, agitated, and can't think clearly. Because she gets annoyed so easily, she feels bad about herself, always guilty.

Like many women, Joan's depression gets worse before her period. Premenstrually, she also gets abdominal distention, craves sweets, and has an increased appetite. Her breasts become sore and painful, especially the nipples. Her emotions fluctuate constantly and she feels extremely irritable, lashing out at the people around her. Her periods have always been irregular, sometimes coming early, sometimes late. She also bleeds excessively once her period does come, sometimes for more than a week. Her blood flow is darker at the beginning and mixed with blood clots. It flows intermittently, stopping and starting.

When I ask to see her tongue, it appears puffy, a bit redder than normal, especially the sides and tip. It trembles, has a deep crack in the center, and white-yellowish fur which is thicker towards the back. Her pulse is bowstring and a bit slippery. It also feels soggy over her wrist bone on the right side.

How a Chinese doctor analyzes Joan's symptoms

Joan's irritability, frustration, wanting to be alone, burping, premenstrual breast distention, and her bowstring pulse all indicate liver depression qi stagnation. Her constant hunger, thirst, dry mouth, and red tongue indicate that this stagnation has transformed into heat which is affecting the stomach. This is corroborated by the especially sensitive and sore nipples premenstrually, a good sign of depressive heat in the liver. Her agitation, restlessness, insomnia, and dream-disturbed sleep indicate that this heat is also disturbing the spirit residing in the heart. Her weight gain, abdominal distention after meals, fatigue, and facial edema as well as the soggy pulse on her right wrist all indicate spleen vacuity or weakness. This is corroborated by increased fatigue when she eats foods which damage the spleen and generate dampness. Because her spleen is weak, dampness and phlegm have accumulated which then obstructs the free flow of qi all the more. When her menses come late, this is because of the liver depression qi stagnation. Her early periods and heavy menstrual bleeding are probably a combination of depressive heat forcing the blood to run frenetically outside its channels and spleen qi vacuity failing to hold the blood within its channels. Based on the clots in her menstruate, there may even be some blood stasis due to long-term qi stagnation.

Because of Joan's constitutional body type, it is likely that her spleen vacuity is, at least in part, constitutional. Everyone is different, including the relative strengths and weaknesses of the viscera and bowels. Some people are born with a weaker spleen than others. However, her depressive episodes have historically been precipitated by specifically psychosocial stressors. In other words, spleen vacuity, even with dampness and phlegm, are not enough to trigger a depressive episode in Joan. It is only when liver depression qi stagnation is aggravated past a certain point that *that* plus the further weakening of the spleen which this inevitably entails results in a depressive episode. Once such an episode gets going, then Joan's diet and behavior either act to keep it going or to lighten it and bring it to an end. In addition, Joan's depression is intimately connected with her menstrual and premenstrual complaints. Remedying of the one would simultaneously improve the other according to Chinese medicine.

If we put this all together, the Chinese doctor knows that there is liver depression with depressive heat harassing above, spleen vacuity with phlegm and dampness gumming up the works, and maybe an element of blood stasis. Whether or not this last element exists is yet to be conclusively decided but may become clear once treatment has been initiated.

How a Chinese doctor treats Joan's depression

Once a Chinese doctor knows the patient's pattern discrimination, the next step is to formulate the treatment principles necessary to rebalance the imbalance implied by this pattern discrimination. If the Chinese doctor listed liver depression transforming heat as the main pattern, then the treatment principles are to course the liver and rectify the qi, clear heat and resolve depression. If the Chinese doctor said that there was spleen vacuity secondarily, then the next principles are to fortify the spleen and boost the qi. If this spleen vacuity has given rise to phlegm and dampness, then they would add the principles of eliminating dampness and transforming phlegm.

59

Once the Chinese doctor has stated the treatment principles, then they know that anything which works to accomplish these principles will be good for the patient. Using these principles, the Chinese doctor can now select various acupuncture points which achieve these effects. They can prescribe Chinese herbal medicinals which embody these principles. They can make recommendations about what to eat and not eat based on these principles. They can make recommendations on life-style changes. And, in short, they can advise the patient on *any and every aspect of their life*, judging whether something either aids the accomplishment of these principles or works against it.

In Chinese medicine, the internal administration of Chinese "herbal" medicinals is the main modality.[10] So let's look at how a Chinese doctor crafts a prescription for Joan. Because the first treatment principles stated for Joan were to course the liver and rectify the qi, clear heat and resolve depression and because the liver depression is complicating a pattern of spleen vacuity with dampness and phlegm, the Chinese doctor knows that he or she should select their guiding formula from the harmonizing the liver and spleen category of formulas. Depending on the textbook, there are 22-28 main categories of formulas in Chinese medicine, each category correlated to a main treatment principle. The category of harmonizing the liver and spleen, is part of a broader category of harmonizing formulas which are used to treat patterns that involve complex processes in different levels of the body, different organs, as well as the presence of hot and cold simultaneously.

---

[10] We've put the word herbal in quotation marks since Chinese medicine is not entirely herbal. Herbs are medicinals made from parts of plants, their roots, bark, stems, leaves, flowers, etc. Chinese medicinals are mostly herbal in nature. However, a percentage of Chinese medicinals also come from the animal and mineral realms. Thus not all Chinese medicinals are, strictly speaking, herbs.

Under this category of formulas, there is one very famous formula which addresses several of the treatment principles we have said are necessary, *Xiao Chao Hu Tang* (Minor Bupleurum Combination/Decoction). This formula can be used for a wide variety of complaints characterized, on the one hand, by liver depression qi stagnation with the presence of heat and, on the other hand, by spleen vacuity giving rise to dampness and phlegm. The Chinese doctor would then modify this prescription to possibly clear even more heat, boost the qi more, eliminate dampness or transform phlegm more, or to address her menstrual complaints more effectively.

If the formula was modified from its textbook or standard form in order to fit the patient more perfectly, the final formula would be called *Xiao Chai Hu Tang Jia Wei* (Minor Bupleurum Decoction with Added Flavors [*i.e.,* ingredients). The standard formula is comprised of:

Radix Bupleuri *(Chai Hu)*
Radix Scutellariae Baicalensis *(Huang Qin)*
Radix Panacis Ginseng *(Ren Shen)*
Rhizoma Pinelliae Ternatae *(Ban Xia)*
mix-fried Radix Glycyrrhizae *(Gan Cao)*
uncooked Rhizoma Zingiberis *(Sheng Jiang)*
Fructus Zizyphi Jujubae *(Da Zao)*

Bupleurum courses the liver and rectifies the qi while scattering internal heat through diaphoresis. Ginseng fortifies the spleen and supplements the qi of the entire organism. It also quiets the spirit. Scutellaria clears heat from the lungs (manifested as uncontrolled crying) and stomach (excessive appetite) as well as from the liver and heart. Pinellia harmonizes or downbears the stomach. It also transforms phlegm and eliminates dampness via the spleen's movement and transformation. Uncooked or fresh ginger, assists pinellia in all of these functions and promotes the movement of qi. Glycyrrhiza or licorice supplements the spleen and heart. It also helps harmonize all the other ingredients in the

61

formula and prevents them from having unwanted side effects. Zizyphus Jujuba or red dates supplement the spleen and nourish the heart. In this formula, they assist ginseng and licorice.

Some of the medicinals which might be added in order to tailor this formula more to Joan's exact needs and condition are Cortex Albizziae Julibrissinis (*He Huan Pi*) to calm her spirit. It is used for insomnia and irritability due to qi stagnation. Radix Polygalae Tenuifoliae (*Yuan Zhi*) both calms the spirit and transforms phlegm. It's very helpful in cases of depression characterized by excessive brooding and disorientation combined with constrained emotions. Rhizoma Acori Graminei (*Shi Chang Pu*) is an aromatic substance which transforms phlegm and "opens the orifices." It is used when phlegm blocks and prevents the clear yang of consciousness. As we saw in the section describing the continuum of phlegm dampness obstruction and stagnation patterns, phlegm confounding the orifices of the heart may cause lassitude of the spirit, lack of clarity of thought, confusion, and excessive rumination.

Usually, a formula such as this when used to treat depression would be taken two to three times each day. The herbs would be soaked in water and then boiled into a very strong "tea" for 30-45 minutes. Each week, the Chinese doctor would check with Joan to see how she was doing and if they needed to make any modifications to her formula. Remember, the practitioner of Chinese medicine wants to heal without causing *any* side effects. If the formula does cause any unwanted effects, then it is the Chinese doctor's job to add and subtract ingredients until the herbs achieve a perfect result with no unwanted effects.

The ingredients in this formula may also be taken as a dried, powdered extract. Such extracts are manufactured by several Taiwanese and Japanese companies. Although such extracts are not, in our experience, as powerful as the freshly decocted "teas", they are easier to take. Many standard formulas also come as ready-made pills. However, these cannot be modified. If their ingredients match the individual patient's requirements, then they are fine. If the formula needs modifications, then teas or powders whose individual ingredients can be added and subtracted are necessary.

In exactly the same way, the practitioner of Chinese medicine could create an individualized acupuncture treatment plan and would certainly create an accompanying dietary and life-style plan. However, we will discuss each of these in their own chapter. In a woman Joan's age with her Chinese pattern discrimination, either Chinese herbal medicine alone, acupuncture alone, or a combination of the two supported by the proper diet and life-style will usually eliminate or at the very least drastically diminish her depression within two to three weeks. Often results will be apparent the first day after taking a full dose of the herbs. However, the reader should understand that such Chinese medicinals are not like antidepressants. Chinese medicinals such as these act to restore balance and harmony to the yin and yang of the body. Therefore, they do not usually provide immediate symptomatic relief for depression, in the same way as taking Prozac does. Conversely, they also do not cause any side effects.

Chinese Herbal Medicine & Depression

As we have seen from Joan's case above, there is no Chinese "anti-depression herb" or even a single "anti-depression formula" which will work for all sufferers of depression. Chinese medicinals are individually prescribed based on a person's pattern discrimination, not on a disease diagnosis like depression. Patients often come to practitioners of Chinese medicine saying, "My friend told me that *Xiao Yao Wan* (Free and Easy Pills, a common Chinese over-the-counter medication) is good for depression. But I tried it and it didn't work." This is because *Xiao Yao Wan* is meant to treat a *specific pattern* of depression, not depression per se. If you exhibit that pattern, then this formula will work. If you do not have signs and symptoms of this pattern, it won't.

In addition, because most people's depression is a combination of different Chinese patterns and disease mechanisms, professional Chinese medicine never treats depression with herbal "singles." In herbalism, singles mean the prescription of a single herb all by itself. Chinese herbal medicine is based on rebalancing patterns, and patterns in real-life patients almost always have more than a single element. Therefore, Chinese doctors almost always prescribe herbs in multi-ingredient formulas. Such formula may have anywhere from 6 to 18 or more ingredients. When a practitioner of Chinese medicine reads a prescription by another practitioner, they can tell you not only what the patient's pattern discrimination is but also their probable signs and symptoms. In other words, the practitioner of Chinese medicine does not just combine several medicinals which are all reputed to be "good for depression." Rather, they carefully craft a formula whose ingredients are meant to rebalance every aspect of the patient's body-mind.

Getting your own individualized prescription

Since, in China, it takes not less than four years of full-time college education to learn how to do a professional Chinese pattern discrimination and then write an herbal formula based on that pattern discrimination, most laypeople cannot realistically write their own Chinese herbal prescriptions. It should also be remembered that Chinese herbs are not effective and safe because they are either Chinese or herbal. In fact, approximately 20% of the common Chinese materia medica did not originate in China, and not all Chinese herbs are completely safe. They are only safe when prescribed according to a correct pattern discrimination, in the right dose, and for the right amount of time. After all, if an herb is strong enough to heal and balance, it is also strong enough to create an imbalance if overdosed or misprescribed. Therefore, we strongly recommend persons who wish to experience the many benefits of Chinese herbal medicine to see a qualified professional practitioner who can do a professional pattern discrimination and write you an individualized prescription. Towards the end of this book, we will give the reader suggestions on how to find a qualified professional Chinese medical practitioner near you.

Experimenting with Chinese patent medicines

In reality, qualified professional practitioners of Chinese medicine are not yet found in every North American community. In addition, some people may want to try to heal their depression as much on their own as possible. More and more health food stores are stocking a variety of ready-made Chinese formulas in pill and powder form. These ready-made, over-the-counter Chinese medicines are often referred to as Chinese patent medicines. Although our best recommendation is for readers to seek Chinese herbal treatment from professional practitioners, below are some suggestions of how one might experiment with Chinese patent medicines to treat depression.

In chapter 5, we have given the signs and symptoms of the seven key or basic patterns associated with most people's depression. These are:

1. Liver depression qi stagnation
2. Liver depression transforms heat
3. Liver blood stasis & stagnation
4. Phlegm dampness obstruction and stagnation
5. Phlegm fire harassing the spirit
6. Anxiety & worry harassing the heart spirit
7. Heart-spleen dual vacuity
8. Spleen-kidney yang vacuity
9. Yin vacuity with fire effulgence

If the reader can identify their main pattern from chapter 5, then there are some Chinese patent remedies that they might consider trying.

Xiao Yao Wan (also spelled *Hsiao Yao Wan*)

Xiao Yao Wan is one of the most common Chinese herbal formulas prescribed. Its Chinese name has been translated as Free & Easy Pills, Rambling Pills, Relaxed Wanderer Pills, and several other versions of this same idea of promoting a freer and smoother, more relaxed flow. As a patent medicine, this formula comes as pills, and there are both Chinese-made and American-made versions of this formula available over the counter in the North American marketplace.[11]

The ingredients in this formula are:

---

[11] When marketed as a dried, powdered extract, this formula is sold under the name of Bupleurum & Tang-kuei Formula.

Radix Bupleuri (*Chai Hu*)
Radix Angelicae Sinensis (*Dang Gui*)
Radix Albus Paeoniae Lactiflorae (*Bai Shao*)
Rhizoma Atractylodis Macrocephalae (*Bai Zhu*)
Sclerotium Poriae Cocos (*Fu Ling*)
mix-fried Radix Glycyrrhizae (*Gan Cao*)
Herba Menthae Haplocalycis (*Bo He*)
uncooked Rhizoma Zingiberis (*Sheng Jiang*)

This formula treats the pattern of liver depression qi stagnation complicated by blood vacuity and spleen weakness with possible dampness as well. Bupleurum courses the liver and rectifies the qi. It is aided in this by Herba Menthae Haplocalycis or mint. Dang Gui and Radix Albus Paeoniae Lactilforae or white peony nourish the blood and soften and harmonize the liver. Rhizoma Atractylodis Macrocephalae or atractylodes and Sclerotium Poriae Cocos or poria fortify the spleen and eliminate dampness. Mix-fried licorice aid these two in fortifying the spleen and supplementing the liver, while uncooked ginger aids in both promoting and regulating the qi flow and eliminating dampness.

When depression presents with the signs and symptoms of liver depression, spleen qi vacuity, and an element of blood vacuity, one can try taking this formula. However, after taking these pills at the dose recommended on the packaging, if one notices any side effects, then stop immediately and seek a professional consultation. Such side effects from this formula might include nervousness, irritability, a dry mouth and increased thirst, and red, dry eyes. Such side effects show that this formula, at least without modification, is not right for you. Although it may be doing you some good, it is also causing some harm. Remember, Chinese medicine is meant to cure without side effects, and as long as the prescription matches one's pattern there will not be any.

Dan Zhi Xiao Yao Wan

Dan Zhi Xiao Yao Wan or Moutan & Gardenia Rambling Pills is a modification of the above formula which also comes as a patent medicine in the form of pills.[12] It is meant to treat the pattern of liver depression transforming into heat with spleen vacuity and possible blood vacuity and/or dampness. The ingredients in this formula are the same as above except that two other herbs are added:

Cortex Radicis Moutan (*Dan Pi*)
Fructus Gardeniae Jasminoidis (*Shan Zhi Zi*)

These two ingredients clear heat and resolve depression. In addition, Cortex Radicis Moutan or moutan quickens the blood and dispels stasis and is good at clearing heat specifically from the blood. Some Chinese doctors say to take out uncooked ginger and mint, while other leave these two ingredients in.

Basically, the signs and symptoms of the pattern for which this formula is designed are the same as those for *Xiao Yao Wan* above plus signs and symptoms of depressive heat. These might include a reddish tongue with slightly yellow fur, a bowstring and rapid pulse, a bitter taste in the mouth, and increased irritability.

Chai Hu Jia Long Gu Mu Li Wan

Chai Hu Jia Long Gu Mu Li Wan or Bupleurum, Dragon Bone & Oyster Shell Pills are the pill form of a formula which has been used in China and other Asian countries for 1,700 years. It is for the treatment of liver depression/depressive heat and spleen vacuity causing mental-emotional anxiety, unrest, insomnia, and heart palpitations. Its ingredients include:

[12] When marketed as a dried, powdered extract, this formula is called Bupleurum & Peony Formula.

69

Radix Bupleuri (*Chai Hu*)
Radix Panacis Ginseng (*Ren Shen*)
Rhizoma Pinelliae Ternatae (*Ban Xia*)
Sclerotium Poriae Cocos (*Fu Ling*)
Ramulus Cinnamomi Cassiae (*Gui Zhi*)
Radix Scutellariae Baicalensis (*Huang Qin*)
Fructus Zizyphi Jujubae (*Da Zao*)
Os Draconis (*Long Gu*)
Concha Ostreae (*Mu Li*)
dry Rhizoma Zingiberis (*Gan Jiang*)
Radix Et Rhizoma Rhei (*Da Huang*)

Because this formula contains rhubarb, this formula is especially effective for those suffering from constipation. If this formula causes diarrhea, its use should be immediately discontinued and professional advice sought.

Chai Hu Shu Gan Wan

Chai Hu Shu Gan Wan means Bupleurum Soothe the Liver Pills. They treat liver depression qi stagnation, the main mechanism of most people's depression. These pills course the liver and rectify the qi, resolve depression and loosen the chest. Their ingredients consist of:

Radix Bupleuri (*Chai Hu*)
Radix Albus Paeoniae Lactiflorae (*Bai Shao*)
Rhizoma Cyperi Rotundi (*Xiang Fu*)
Fructus Citri Aurantii (*Zhi Ke*)
Radix Ligustici Wallichii (*Chuan Xiong*)
Radix Glycyrrhizae (*Gan Cao*)

Unlike the preceding formulas, this one does not contain any ingredients which fortify the spleen and supplement the qi. It is completely focused on moving and rectifying the qi.

70

Da Chai Hu Wan

Meaning Great Bupleurum Pills, this formula is for rather severe liver depression of recent onset or in a robust, strong con-stitutioned person with a tendency to constipation. It courses the liver and rectifies the qi, clears heat and frees the flow of the stools. Its ingredients consist of:

Radix Bupleuri (*Chai Hu*)
Rhizoma Pinelliae Ternatae (*Ban Xia*)
Radix Scutellariae Baicalensis (*Huang Qin*)
Fructus Citri Aurantii (*Zhi Ke*)
Radix Albus Paeoniae Lactiflorae (*Bai Shao*)
dry Rhizoma Zingiberis (*Gan Jiang*)
Fructus Zizyphi Jujubae (*Da Zao*)
Radix Et Rhizoma Rhei (*Da Huang*)

Like Bupleurum, Dragon Bone & Oyster Shell Pills above, because this formula contains rhubarb, it is especially useful for those with constipation with dry, hard, bound stools. If this formula causes diarrhea, it should be suspended immediately.

Xiao Chai Hu Wan

If *Da Chai Hu Wan* means Great Bupleurum Pills, then *Xiao Chai Hu Wan* means Small or Minor Bupleurum Pills. This formula is also for liver depression/depressive heat. However, it is indicated for those with concomitant spleen vacuity and no constipation. In fact, it is a good formula for those with a tendency to soft or loose stools. This is the pill formula of the prescription given to Joan in the preceding chapter. It is the most commonly prescribed Chinese herbal formula in the world with a wide range of indications. It is called a harmonizing formula since it harmonizes the inside and outside of the body, the liver and spleen, the spleen and stomach, and the stomach and intestines. Its ingredients consist of:

Radix Bupleuri (*Chai Hu*)

71

Rhizoma Pinelliae Ternatae (*Ban Xia*)
Radix Codonopsitis Pilosulae (*Dang Shen*)
Radix Scutellariae Baicalensis (*Huang Qin*)
Fructus Zizyphi Jujubae (*Da Zao*)
Radix Glycyrrhizae (*Gan Cao*)
dry Rhizoma Zingiberis (*Gan Jiang*)

Shu Gan Wan

The name of this formula means Soothe the Liver Pills. In English, these pills are erroneously identified as Hepatic Tonic Pills. They primarily course the liver and rectify the qi. They are especially recommended when stagnant qi affects digestion and is accompanied by upper abdominal and hypochondral pain and distention. Their ingredients are:

Fructus Meliae Toosendan (*Chuan Lian Zi*)
Rhizoma Curcumae Longae (*Jiang Huang*)
Lignum Aquilariae Agallochae (*Chen Xiang*)
Rhizoma Corydalis Yanhusuo (*Yan Hu Suo*)
Radix Auklandiae Lappae (*Mu Xiang*)
Semen Mrysticae Fragrantis (*Dou Kou*)
Radix Albus Paeoniae Lactiflorae (*Bai Shao*)
Sclerotium Poriae Cocos (*Fu Ling*)
Fructus Citri Aurantii (*Zhi Ke*)
Pericarpium Citri Reticulatae (*Chen Pi*)
Fructus Amomi (*Sha Ren*)
Cortex Magnoliae Officinalis (*Huo Po*)

A condensed version of the same formula sold as *Shu Kan Wan*, more effectively moves liver depression qi stagnation. It deletes Fructus Meliae Toosendan and Sclerotium Poriae Cocos and adds eight additional herbs:

Rhizoma Cyperi Rotundi (*Xiang Fu*)
Radix Glycyrrhizae (*Gan Cao*)
Cortex Radicis Moutan (*Dan Pi*)

72

Radix Bupleuri (*Chai Hu*)
Fructus Citri Sacrodactylis (*Fo Shou*)
Pericarpium Citri Reticulatae Viride (*Qing Pi*)
Fructus Citri Medicae (*Xiang Yuan*)
Lignum Santalli Albi (*Tan Xiang*)

Mu Xiang Shun Qi Wan

The name of this formula translates as Auklandia Normalize the Qi Pills. It courses the liver and rectifies the qi. It is also recommended in cases of qi stagnation affecting the digestion and causing food stagnation. It relieves abdominal pain, boosts the stomach, and disperses food accumulation. It is used to treat feelings of fullness in the chest, diaphragm, and hypochondrium. Its ingredients are:

Radix Auklandia Lappae (*Mu Xiang*)
Semen Myrsticae Fragrantis (*Dou Kou*)
Rhizoma Atractylodis (*Cang Zhu*)
uncooked Rhizoma Zingiberis (*Sheng Jiang*)
Pericarpium Citri Reticulatae Viride (*Qing Pi*)
Pericarpium Citri Reticulatae (*Chen Pi*)
Sclerotium Poriae Cocos (*Fu Ling*)
Radix Bupleuri (*Chai Hu*)
Cortex Magnoliae Officinalis (*Hou Po*)
Semen Arecae Catechu (*Bing Lang*)
Fructus Citri Aurantii (*Zhi Ke*)
Radix Linderae Strychnifoliae (*Wu Yao*)
Semen Raphani Sativi (*Lai Fu Zi*)
Fructus Crataegi (*Shan Zha*)
Massa Medica Fermentata (*Shen Qu*)
Fructus Germinatus Hordei Vulgaris (*Mai Ya*)
Radix Glycyrrhizae (*Gan Cao*)

Gan Mai Da Zao Wan

The name of these pills translates as Licorice, Wheat & Red Dates Pills. This formula is specifically for the pattern of depression known as depression and anxiety harassing the heart. This is a combination of liver depression and heart qi vacuity resulting in restlessness and agitation, alternating tendencies to euphoria and tears, and the possibility of night sweats. This small formula can be added to a number of other formulas when either alternating euphoria and tears or night sweats complicate other conditions. The ingredients in this formula are:

Fructus Levis Tritici Aestivi (*Fu Xiao Mai*)
Radix Glycyrrhizae (*Gan Cao*)
Fructus Zizyphi Jujubae (*Da Zao*)
Bulbus Lilii (*Bai He*)
Cortex Albizziae Julibrissinis (*He Huan Pi*)
Radix Polygoni Multiflori (*He Shou Wu*)
Sclerotium Poriae Cocos (*Fu Ling*)

This formula can be especially effective for women's pre-menstrual and perimenopausal depression and anxiety. If there are night sweats, for sure it should be tried. It is quite a safe formula. However, because it contains licorice and licorice can raise the blood pressure, those with high blood pressure should probably not use these pills. The good news is that most women with this condition tend to have lower than normal blood pressure.

An Shen Yang Xin Cha

Marketed under the English name Shen Classic Tea, these prepackaged tea bags are meant for heart qi and blood vacuity with an element of liver depression. They can be drunk as a daily beverage for those with mental-emotional restlessness and anxiety, insomnia and heart palpitations due to heart qi and blood vacuity. They are not meant for these same conditions when due to pathological heat or phlegm. Their ingredients consist of:

74

Folium Mori Albi (*Sang Ye*)
Sclerotium Poriae Cocos (*Fu Ling*)
Radix Polygoni Multiflori (*He Shou Wu*)
Radix Salviae Miltiorrhizae (*Dan Shen*)
Radix Polygalae Tenuifoliae (*Yuan Zhi*)

Gui Pi Wan (also spelled *Kuei Pi Wan*)

Gui means to return or restore, *pi* means the spleen, and *wan* means pills. Therefore, the name of these pills means Restore the Spleen Pills.[13] However, these pills not only supplement the spleen qi but also nourish heart blood and calm the heart spirit. They are the textbook guiding formula for the pattern of heart-spleen dual vacuity. In this case, there are symptoms of spleen qi vacuity, such as fatigue, poor appetite, and cold hands and feet plus symptoms of heart blood vacuity, such as a pale tongue, heart palpitations, and insomnia. This formula is also the standard one for treating heavy or abnormal bleeding due to the spleen not containing and restraining the blood within its vessels. Therefore, this patent medicine can be combined with *Xiao Yao San* when there is liver depression qi stagnation complicated by heart blood and spleen qi vacuity. Its ingredients are:

Radix Astragali Membranacei (*Huang Qi*)
Radix Codonopsitis Pilosulae (*Dang Shen*)
Rhizoma Atractylodis Macrocephalae (*Bai Zhu*)
Sclerotium Pararadicis Poriae Cocos (*Fu Shen*)
mix-fried Radix Glycyrrhizae (*Gan Cao*)
Radix Angelicae Sinensis (*Dang Gui*)
Semen Zizyphi Spinosae (*Suan Zao Ren*)
Arillus Euphoriae Longanae (*Long Yan Rou*)
Radix Polygalae Tenuifoliae (*Yuan Zhi*)
Radix Auklandiae Lappae (*Mu Xiang*)

---

[13] When sold as a dried, powdered extract, this formula is called Ginseng & Longan Combination.

Er Chen Wan

Er Chen Wan means Two Aged (Ingredients) Pills.[14] This is because, two of its main ingredients are aged before using. This formula is used to transform phlegm and eliminate dampness. It can be added to *Xiao Yao Wan* if there is liver depression with spleen vacuity and more pronounced phlegm and dampness. If there is liver depression transforming heat giving rise to phlegm heat, it can be combined with *Dan Zhi Xiao Yao Wan*. Its ingredients include:

Rhizoma Pinelliae Ternatae (*Ban Xia*)
Sclerotium Poriae Cocos (*Fu Ling*)
mix-fried Radix Glycyrrhizae (*Gan Cao*)
Pericarpium Citri Reticulatae (*Chen Pi*)
uncooked Rhizoma Zingiberis (*Sheng Jiang*)

Su Zi Jiang Qi Wan

Su Zi is the name of a Chinese herb, Perilla seeds. *Jiang qi* means to downbear the qi. Therefore, the name of this patent medicine means Perilla Seed Downbear the Qi Pills. This patent formula is usually prescribed for asthma, shortness of breath, and cough. But because it transforms phlegm, downbears counterflow, and regulates the stomach qi, it can be helpful in the treatment of depression due to phlegm dampness obstruction and stagnation, especially if combined with *Xiao Yao San* in order to treat the typically accompanying liver depression qi stagnation. Its ingredients are:

Fructus Perillae Frutescentis (*Su Zi*)
Rhizoma Pinelliae Ternatae (*Ban Xia*)
Cortex Magnoliae Officinalis (*Huo Po*)
Radix Peucedani (*Qian Hu*)

---

[14] When sold as a dried, powdered extract, this formula is called Citrus & Pinellia Combination.

Pericarpium Citri Reticulatae (*Chen Pi*)
Lignum Aquilariae Agallochae (*Chen Xiang*)
Radix Angelicae Sinensis (*Dang Gui*)
uncooked Rhizoma Zingiberis (*Sheng Jiang*)
Fructus Zizyphi Jujubae (*Da Zao*)
Radix Glycyrrhizae (*Gan Cao*)

Liu Wei Di Huang Wan

This formula, whose name means Six Flavors Rehmannia Pills, nourishes liver blood and kidney yin. It is the primary formula to treat symptoms of yin vacuity. It can be combined with other patent medicines in cases of depression with a strong component of yin vacuity, such as is commonly encountered around menopause or in older people. For instance, these pills can be combined with *Xiao Yao Wan* or even *Dan Zhi Xiao Yao Wan*. Its ingredients are:

cooked Radix Rehmanniae (*Shu Di*)
Fructus Corni Officinalis (*Shan Zhu Yu*)
Radix Dioscoreae Oppositae (*Shan Yao*)
Rhizoma Alismatis (*Ze Xie*)
Sclerotium Poriae Cocos (*Fu Ling*)
Cortex Radicis Moutan (*Dan Pi*)

If there are signs and symptoms of vacuity heat, then another formula should be used instead. It is made by adding two more ingredients to the above:

Rhizoma Anemarrhenae Aspheloidis (*Zhi Mu*)
Cortex Phellodendri (*Huang Bai*)

This is then called *Zhi Bai Di Huang Wan*, Anemarrhena & Phellodendron Rehmannia Pills. For instance, a very commonly prescribed combination is *Zhi Bai Di Huang Wan* and *Bu Zhong Yi Qi Wan* described below for spleen qi vacuity, liver depression, kidney yin vacuity, and yin vacuity and/or damp heat, *i.e.*, the complex yin fire scenario we talked about above.

77

Jin Gui Shen Qi Wan

The name of these commonly available Chinese patent pills translates as Golden Cabinet Kidney Qi Pills. The golden cabinet is an allusion to the name of the book this formula is first recorded in, the *Jin Gui Yao Lue (Essentials from the Golden Cabinet)* dating from 200-250 CE. This is the most famous formula for the treatment of kidney yang vacuity, and it can be combined with other formulas when kidney yang vacuity complicates a patient's pattern discrimination. Its ingredients include:

cooked Radix Rehmanniae (*Shu Di*)
Fructus Corni Officinalis (*Shan Zhu Yu*)
Radix Dioscoreae Oppositae (*Shan Yao*)
Sclerotium Poriae Cocos (*Fu Ling*)
Rhizoma Alismatis (*Ze Xie*)
Cortex Radicis Moutan (*Dan Pi*)
Radix Lateralis Praeparatus Aconiti Carmichaeli (*Fu Zi*)
Cortex Cinnamomi Cassiae (*Rou Gui*)

Because this formula contains at least two very hot herbs, one should not take this formula if they have any signs or symptoms of heat or they should get a diagnosis and prescription for this formula from a professional practitioner.

Tian Wang Bu Xin Dan

The name of this formula translates as Heavenly Emperor's Supplement the Heart Elixir.[15] This formula comes as a Chinese patent medicine in pill form. It treats insomnia, restlessness, fatigue, and heart palpitations due to yin, blood, and qi vacuity, with an emphasis on heart yin and liver blood vacuity. Its ingredients include:

---

[15] When marketed as a desiccated, powdered extract, this formula is sold under the name Ginseng and Zizyphus Formula.

uncooked Radix Rehmanniae (*Sheng Di*)
Radix Scrophulariae Ningpoensis (*Xuan Shen*)
Fructus Schisandrae Chinensis (*Wu Wei Zi*)
Tuber Asparagi Cochinensis (*Tian Men Dong*)
Tuber Ophiopogonis Japonici (*Mai Men Dong*)
Radix Angelicae Sinensis (*Dang Gui*)
Semen Biotae Orientalis (*Bai Zi Ren*)
Semen Zizyphi Spinosae (*Suan Zao Ren*)
Radix Salviae Miltiorrhizae (*Dan Shen*)
Radix Polygalae Tenuifoliae (*Yuan Zhi*)
Sclerotium Poriae Cocos (*Fu Ling*)
Radix Codonopsitis Pilosulae (*Dang Shen*)

Bai Zi Yang Xin Wan (also spelled *Pai Tsu Yang Hsin Wan*)

The name of this formula translates as Biota Seed Nourish the Heart Pills. This is another commonly used over-the-counter Chinese patent pill. It is usually marketed for insomnia, but it can be helpful when depression is characterized by heart yin and liver blood vacuity complicated by an element of phlegm obstruction. If liver depression qi stagnation or liver depression transforming heat complicate the scenario, this formula can be combined with *Xiao Yao Wan* or *Dan Zhi Xiao Yao Wan* respectively. Its ingredients include:

Semen Biotae Orientalis (*Bai Zi Ren*)
Fructus Lycii Chinensis (*Gou Qi Zi*)
Radix Scrophulariae Ningpoensis (*Xuan Shen*)
uncooked Radix Rehmanniae (*Sheng Di*)
Tuber Ophiopogonis Japonici (*Mai Men Dong*)
Radix Angelicae Sinensis (*Dang Gui*)
Sclerotium Poriae Cocos (*Fu Ling*)
Rhizoma Acori Graminei (*Shi Chang Pu*)
Radix Glycyrrhizae (*Gan Cao*)

Tabellae *Suan Zao Ren Tang*

This is the tableted form of a famous spirit-calming Chinese medicinal decoction, Zizyphus Spinosa Decoction. Its ingredients are:

Semen Zizyphi Spinosae (*Suan Zao Ren*)
Radix Ligustici Wallichii (*Chuan Xiong*)
Sclerotium Poriae Cocos (*Fu Ling*)
Rhizoma Anemarrhenae Aspheloidis (*Zhi Mu*)
Radix Glycyrrhizae (*Gan Cao*)

This formula is for insomnia and restlessness or anxiety due primarily to liver blood vacuity with possibly a little heat disturbing the heart spirit. It can be added to any of the liver depression formulas suggested above.

Ding Xin Wan

The name of this Chinese patent pill translates as Stabilize the Heart Pills. It supplements the heart qi and blood, quiets the heart spirit, and clears heat disturbing the heart from the liver and/or stomach. It can be taken in combination with liver depression and transformative heat formulas described above where heart qi and blood vacuity with transformative heat leads to restless spirit, anxiety, heart palpitations, and insomnia. Its ingredients include:

Radix Codonopsitis Pilosulae (*Dang Shen*)
Radix Angelicae Sinensis (*Dang Gui*)
Sclerotium Pararadicis Poriae Cocos (*Fu Shen*)
Radix Polygalae Tenuifoliae (*Yuan Zhi*)
Semen Zizyphi Spinosae (*Suan Zao Ren*)
Semen Biotae Orientalis (*Bai Zi Ren*)
Radix Scutellariae Baicalensis (*Huang Qin*)
Tuber Ophiopogonis Japonici (*Mai Men Dong*)
Succinum (*Hu Po*)

80

An Mian Pian

These are called Quiet Sleep Pills. They can be used by themselves or combined with other appropriate patent pills for insomnia and restlessness due to liver depression transforming heat and liver blood not nourishing the heart spirit. Their ingredients are:

Semen Zizyphi Spinosae (*Suan Zao Ren*)
Radix Polygalae Tenuifoliae (*Yuan Zhi*)
Sclerotium Poriae Cocos (*Fu Ling*)
Fructus Gardeniae Jasminoidis (*Shan Zhi Zi*)
Massa Medica Fermentata (*Shen Qu*)
Radix Glycyrrhizae (*Gan Cao*)

Tong Jing Wan (also spelled To Jing Wan)

The name of these pills means Painful Menstruation Pills. Depression is often complicated by blood stasis in women and the elderly. The symptoms of blood stasis include painful menstruation with the passage of dark clots, pain which is stabbing or intense in nature and tends to be fixed in position, a dark, dusky facial complexion, possible black circles under the eyes, purplish lips, a purplish tongue, possible static blood patches or dots on the tongue, spider nevi, small, red hemangiomas, varicosities, hemorrhoids, or thrombophlebitis, and a bowstring, choppy pulse.[16] In such cases, this pill can be taken along with other appropriate formulas when blood stasis is an important factor in someone's depression. Its ingredients are:

Tuber Curcumae (*Yu Jin*)
Rhizoma Sparganii (*San Leng*)
Radix Rubrus Paeoniae Lactiflorae (*Chi Shao*)
Radix Angelicae Sinensis (*Dang Gui*)

---

[16] A choppy pulse is a fine, somewhat slow pulse which tends to speed up and slow down (often with the breathing) but does not necessarily skip any beats.

81

Radix Ligustici Wallichii (*Chuan Xiong*)
Radix Salviae Miltiorrhizae (*Dan Shen*)
Flos Carthami Tinctorii (*Hong Hua*)

Xue Fu Zhu Yu Wan

The name of these pills means Blood Mansion Dispel Stasis Pills. They are yet another Chinese patent medicine in pill form for the treatment of blood stasis. This formula is the one that Wu and Bai suggest for liver blood stasis and stagnation emotional depression. Its ingredients include:

Semen Pruni Persicae (*Tao Ren*)
Radix Angelicae Sinensis (*Dang Gui*)
Flos Carthami Tinctorii (*Hong Hua*)
uncooked Radix Rehmanniae (*Sheng Di*)
Radix Achyranthis Bidentatae (*Niu Xi*)
Radix Ligustici Wallichii (*Chuan Xiong*)
Radix Rubrus Paeoniae Lactiflorae (*Chi Shao*)
Fructus Citri Aurantii (*Zhi Ke*)
Radix Bupleuri (*Chai Hu*)
Radix Platycodi Grandiflori (*Jie Geng*)
Radix Glycyrrhizae (*Gan Cao*)

Bu Zhong Yi Qi Wan

The name of this formula translates as Supplement the Center & Boost the Qi Decoction. It strongly supplements spleen vacuity. It is commonly used to treat central qi fall, *i.e.*, prolapse of the stomach, uterus, or rectum due to spleen qi vacuity. However, it is a very complex formula with a very wide range of indications. It supplements the spleen but also courses the liver and rectifies the qi. It is one of the most commonly prescribed of all Chinese herbal formulas and these pills can be combined with a number of others when spleen qi vacuity and liver depression play a significant role in someone's depression, however without significant blood vacuity or particular dampness. Its ingredients are:

Radix Astragali Membranacei (*Huang Qi*)
Radix Panacis Ginseng (*Ren Shen*)
Radix Glycyrrhizae (*Gan Cao*)
Rhizoma Atractylodis Macrocephalae (*Bai Zhu*)
Radix Angelicae Sinensis (*Dang Gui*)
Pericarpium Citri Reticulatae (*Chen Pi*)
Rhizoma Cimicifugae (*Sheng Ma*)
Radix Bupleuri (*Chai Hu)*
Rhizoma Atractylodis Macrocephalae (*Bai Zhu*)

The above are only the most famous and commonly used formulas which are currently available over the counter at American health food stores and at Asian specialty food stores in Asian communities in North America. They can be ordered by phone, fax, or mail from:

Mayway Corp.
1338 Mandela Parkway
Oakland, CA 94607
Tel. 510-208-3113
Orders: 1-800-2-Mayway
Fax: 510-208-3069
Orders by fax: 1-800-909-2828

This company is one of the largest importers and distributors of Chinese herbs and Chinese herbal products in North America and Europe. They have a very nice, easy to use catalog with easy ordering numbers so you do not need to worry about pronouncing the Chinese names of these formulas.

There are many other important formulas used in the professional practice of Chinese medicine. However, for these, you will need to see your local professional practitioner. If you experiment with Chinese herbal patent medicines for your depression, please be careful. Be sure to follow the six guideposts for assessing the safety of any medications you take.

Six guideposts for assessing any over-the-counter medication

In general, you can tell if *any* medication and treatment are good for you by checking the following six guideposts:

1. Digestion
2. Elimination
3. Energy level

4. Mood
5. Appetite
6. Sleep

If a medication, be it modern Western or traditional Chinese, gets rid of your symptoms and all six of these basic areas of human health improve, then that medicine or treatment is probably OK. However, even if a treatment or medication takes away your major complaint, *if it causes deterioration in any one of these six basic parameters,* then that treatment or medication is probably not OK and is certainly not OK for long-term use. When medicines and treatments, even so-called natural, herbal medications, are prescribed based on a person's pattern of disharmony, then there is healing without side effects. According to Chinese medicine, this is the only kind of true healing.

84

Acupuncture & Moxibustion

Acupuncture is the best known of the various methods of treatment which go to make up Chinese medicine. When the average Westerner thinks of Chinese medicine, they probably first think of acupuncture. In China, acupuncture is actually a secondary treatment modality. Most Chinese immediately think of herbal medicine when they think of Chinese medicine. Nevertheless, depression responds very well to correctly prescribed and administered acupuncture.

What is acupuncture?

Acupuncture primarily means the insertion of extremely thin, sterilized, stainless steel needles into specific points on the body where practitioners of Chinese medicine have known for centuries there are special concentrations of qi and blood. Therefore, these points are like switches or circuit breakers for regulating and balancing the flow of qi and blood over the channel and network system we described above.

As we have seen, depressive episodes are generally the result of an obstruction in the smooth flow of qi and a breakdown in the harmony between the body's yin and yang. The pattern recognized in Chinese medicine as liver depression qi stagnation is intimately connected with the mechanism behind depressive episodes. Liver depression means that the qi is stagnant. Because the qi is depressed and stagnant, it is not flowing when and where it should. Instead it deprives the regions of the body irrigated by the corresponding channels, it counterflows upward, or it vents itself to areas of the body where it shouldn't be, attacking other organs and body tissues and making them dysfunction. Therefore, the Chinese patterns that correspond to depression typically include many signs and symptoms associated with lack of or erroneous qi flow. Since acupuncture's forte is the regulation and rectification of the flow of qi, it is an especially good treatment mode for correcting depression. In that case, insertion of acupuncture needles at various points in the body moves stagnant qi in the liver and leads the qi to flow in its proper directions and amounts.

As a generic term, acupuncture also includes several other methods of stimulating acupuncture points, thus regulating the flow of qi in the body. The main other modality is moxibustion. This means the warming of acupuncture points mainly by burning dried, aged Oriental mugwort on, near, or over acupuncture points. The purpose of this warming treatment are to 1) even more strongly stimulate the flow of qi and blood, 2) add warmth to areas of the body which are too cold, and 3) add yang qi to the body to supplement a yang qi deficiency. Other acupuncture modalities are to apply suction cups over points, to massage the points, to prick the points to allow a drop or two of blood to exit, to apply Chinese medicinals to the points, to apply magnets to the points, and to stimulate the points by either electricity or laser.

What is a typical acupuncture treatment for depression like?

In China, acupuncture treatments are given every day or every other day, three to five times per week depending on the nature and severity of the condition. In the West however, health care delivery differs greatly from China, making it financially unfeasible for most patients to receive as many treatments per week. Western patients suffering from depression respond very well to acupuncture treatment performed twice a week for the first few weeks, following up with treatment every week. In acute depressive episodes, after the initial course of 10-12 sessions, it is best to continue acupuncture treatment weekly for one more month, then tapering gradually to twice a month. After that, a maintenance course of monthly sessions is highly recommended, since depression tends to be a recurrent condition. In chronic, insidious, and severe depressions, acupuncture treatment should continue for several months. In general, one can expect their improvement from acupuncture to be gradual and progressive. Based on our clinical experience, if acupuncture is combined with diet and life-style changes, Chinese herbs, and a selection of the self-care treatments recommended below, the results will be even quicker and the relief of symptoms even more complete.

When the person comes for their appointment, the practitioner will ask them what their main symptoms are, will typically look at their tongue and its fur, and will feel the pulses at the radial arteries on both wrists. Then, they will ask the patient to lie down on a treatment table and may palpate their abdomen and the zones traversed by the different channels to feel for areas of constriction, tenderness, and blockage. Based on the patient's pattern discrimination, the practitioner will select anywhere from one to eight or nine points to be needled.

The needles used today are ethylene oxide gas sterilized disposable needles. This means that they are used one time and then thrown away, just like a hypodermic syringe in a doctor's office. However, unlike relatively fat hypodermic needles, acupuncture needles are hardly thicker than a strand of hair. The skin over the point is disinfected with alcohol and the needle is quickly and deftly inserted somewhere typically between one quarter and a half inch. In some few cases, a needle may be inserted deeper than that, but most needles are only inserted relatively shallowly.

After the needle has broken the skin, the acupuncturist will usually manipulate the needle in various ways until he or she feels that the qi has "arrived." This refers to a subtle but very real feeling of resistance around the needle. When the qi arrives, the patient will usually feel a mild, dull soreness around the needle, a slight electrical feeling, a heavy feeling, or a numb or tingly feeling. All these mean that the needle has tapped the qi and that treatment will be effective. Once the qi has been tapped, then the practitioner may further adjust the qi flow by manipulating the needle in certain ways, may simply leave the needle in place, usually for 10-20 minutes, or may attach the needle to an electro-acupuncture machine in order to stimulate the point with very mild and gentle electricity. After this, the needles are withdrawn and thrown away. *Thus there is absolutely no chance for infection from another patient.*

How are the points selected?

The points one's acupuncturist chooses to needle each treatment are selected on the basis of Chinese medical theory and the known clinical effects of certain points. Since there are different schools or styles of acupuncture, point selection tends to vary from practitioner to practitioner. However, below we present a fairly typical case of acupuncture treatment for depression based on Chinese medical pattern discrimination.

Let's take the case of Joan who we saw before. Her main complaints are irritability, increased appetite and weight gain, lethargy and apathy, and difficulty sleeping. We previously established that Joan's Chinese pattern discrimination is liver depression transforming heat which is then harassing the stomach and heart complicated by dampness and phlegm due to spleen qi vacuity. This is a very commonly encountered Chinese pattern of disharmony in women with depression in their late 20s and early 30s.

The treatment principles necessary for remedying this case are to course the liver and rectify the qi, clear heat and resolve depression, fortify the spleen and boost the qi, eliminate dampness and transform phlegm, and quiet her spirit. In order to accomplish these aims, the practitioner might select the following points:

Tai Chong (Liver 3)
He Gu (Large Intestine 4)
San Yin Jiao (Spleen 6)
Shen Men (Heart 7)
Nei Guan (Pericardium 6)

Jiu Wei (Conception Vessel 15)
Feng Long (Stomach 40)
Shen Ting (Governing Vessel 24)
Ben Shen (Gallbladder 20)

In this case, *Tai Chong* courses the liver and resolves depression, moves and rectifies the qi. Since liver depression qi stagnation is a main disease mechanism either causing or contributing to this woman's depression, this is a main or ruling point in this treatment. Since this woman's easy anger or irritability stems from liver depression, this point also eliminates the source of this woman's vexation.

He Gu is a widely used point with a variety of indications depending on how it is used and with what points it is combined. *He Gu and Tai Chong* combined are known as "the four gates." They are used to free the flow in the entire body and to promote the upbearing of the clear and downbearing of the turbid by the qi mechanism. When used together, these points have a strong effect in relieving qi stagnation. In addition, *He Gu* clears heat from the upper part of the body.

San Yin Jiao is chosen to further course the liver at the same time it fortifies the spleen. It does both these things because both the liver and spleen channels cross at these points.

Shen Men is a point on the heart channel which supplements the heart, clears heat from the heart, and quiets the heart spirit.

Nei Guan is a point on the pericardium channel which frees the flow of qi in the liver and the chest at the same time as it quiets the spirit in the heart. These two points, *Shen Men* and *Nei Guan*, are routinely used for the treatment of various patterns of depression.

Jiu Wei is a point on the conception vessel located just under the diaphragm. It is very helpful in opening depression when that depression manifests as chest oppression. It is also very helpful in calming the spirit.

Feng Long is a point on the stomach channel. Because the spleen and stomach share a mutual interior/exterior relationship, stimulating *Feng Long* can fortify the spleen with yang qi from the stomach which has plenty to spare. In addition, the stomach channel traverses the chest, and, therefore, needling this point can regulate the qi in the chest. In addition, *Feng Long* helps the spleen transform phlegm and dampness.

Shen Ting is a point on the governing vessel which helps quiet the spirit, open the orifices, and arouse the brain, while *Ben Shen* is a point on the gallbladder channel which courses the liver and opens depression. When these two points are used together, they are a very effective combination for treating depression due to liver depression qi stagnation.

Therefore, this combination of nine points addresses Joan's Chinese pattern discrimination *and* her major complaints of depression, insomnia, irritability, fatigue, apathy, and excessive appetite. It remedies both the underlying disease mechanism and addresses certain key symptoms in a very direct and immediate way. Hence it provides symptomatic relief *at the same time as* it corrects the underlying mechanisms of these symptoms.

Does acupuncture hurt?

In Chinese, it is said that acupuncture is *bu tong*, painless. However, most patients will feel soreness, heaviness, electrical tingling, or distention. When done well and sensitively, it should not be sharp, biting, burning, or really painful.

How quickly will I feel the result?

One of the best things about the acupuncture treatment of depression is that its effects are often immediate. Since many of the mechanisms of depression have to do with stuck qi, as soon as the qi is made to flow, the symptoms disappear. Therefore, many patients begin to feel better after the very first treatment.

In addition, because irritability and nervous tension are also mostly due to liver depression qi stagnation, most people will feel an immediate relief of irritability and tension while still on the table. Typically, one will feel a pronounced tranquility and relaxation within five to ten minutes of the insertion of the needles. Many patients do drop off to sleep for a few minutes while the needles are in place.

Who should get acupuncture?

Since most professional practitioners in the West are legally entitled to practice under various acupuncture laws, most acupuncturists will routinely do acupuncture on every patient. Since acupuncture's effects on depression are usually relatively immediate, this is usually a good thing for sufferers of depression. However, acupuncture is particularly effective for liver depression qi stagnation, liver depression transforming heat, and blood stasis patterns of depression.

When a person's depression mostly has to do with qi vacuity, blood vacuity, or yin vacuity, then acupuncture is most effective when combined with internally administered Chinese herbal medicinals. Although moxibustion can add yang qi to the body, acupuncture needles cannot add qi, blood, or yin to a body in short supply of these. The best acupuncture can do in these cases is to stimulate the various viscera and bowels which engender and transform the qi, blood, and yin. Chinese herbs, on the other hand, can directly introduce qi, blood, and yin into the body, thus supplementing vacuities and insufficiencies of these. In cases of depression, where qi, blood, and yin vacuities are pronounced, one should use acupuncture in combination with Chinese medicinals.

Ear acupuncture

Acupuncturists believe there is a map of the entire body in the ear and that by stimulating the corresponding points in the ear, one can remedy those areas and functions of the body. Therefore, many acupuncturists will not only needle points on the body at large but also select one or more points on the ear. In terms of depression, needling the point *Shen Men* (Spirit Gate) can have a profound effect on relaxing tension and irritability and also improving sleep. There are also other points, such as the Sympathetic Point, the Brain Point, and the Subcortex Point which can be very effective in the treatment of depression.

The nice thing about ear acupuncture points is that one can use tiny "press needles" which are shaped like miniature thumb-tacks. These are pressed into the points, covered with adhesive tape, and left in place for five to seven days. This method can provide continuous treatment between regularly scheduled office visits. Thus ear acupuncture is a nice way of extending the duration of an acupuncture treatment. In addition, these ear points can also be stimulated with small metal pellets, radish seeds, or tiny magnets, thus getting the benefits of stimulating these points without having to insert actual needles.

The Three Free Therapies

Although one can experiment cautiously with Chinese herbal medicinals, one cannot really do acupuncture on oneself. Therefore, Chinese herbal medicine and acupuncture and its related modalities mostly require the aid of a professional practitioner. However, there are three free therapies which are crucial to treating depression. These are diet, exercise, and deep relaxation. Only you can take care of these three factors in your health!

Diet

In Chinese medicine, the function of the spleen and stomach are likened to a pot on a stove or still. The stomach receives the foods and liquids which then "rotten and ripen" like a mash in a fermentation vat. The spleen then cooks this mash and drives off (*i.e.,* transforms and upbears) the pure part. This pure part collects in the lungs to become the qi and in the heart to become the blood. In addition, Chinese medicine characterizes this transformation as a process of yang qi transforming yin substance. All the principles of Chinese dietary therapy, including what persons with depression should and should not eat, are derived from these basic "facts."

We have already seen that the spleen is the root of qi and blood engenderment and transformation. Based on this fact, a healthy, strong spleen prevents and treats depression in four ways. First of all, fatigue is *always* a symptom of qi vacuity. Secondly, if the spleen is healthy and strong, it will create sufficient qi to push the blood and move body fluids. Therefore, a sufficiency of pushing or moving spleen qi helps counterbalance or control any tendency of the liver to constrict or constrain the qi flow. Thus, in Chinese medicine, a healthy spleen helps keep the liver in check and free from depression and stagnation. Third, since the spleen is the root of blood production and it is yin blood which keeps yang qi in check, a healthy, strong spleen manufacturing abundant blood insures a sufficiency of heart blood to nourish and quiet the spirit. And fourth, since any qi, but especially blood, remaining unused at the end of the day can be converted into essence during sleep at night, a strong, healthy spleen manufacturing abundant qi and blood also helps insure the bolstering and supplementation of yin by acquired essence.

Therefore, when it comes to Chinese dietary therapy and depression, the fundamental principle is to avoid foods which damage the spleen. Such foods also typically produce dampness and phlegm.

Foods which damage the spleen

In terms of foods which damage the spleen, Chinese medicine begins with uncooked, chilled foods. If the process of digestion is likened to cooking, then cooking is nothing other than predigestion outside of the body. In Chinese medicine, it is a given that the overwhelming majority of all food should be cooked, i.e., predigested. Although cooking may destroy some vital nutrients (in Chinese, qi), cooking does render the remaining nutrients much more easily assimilable. Therefore, even though some nutrients have been lost, the net absorption of nutrients is greater with cooked foods than raw. Further, eating raw foods makes the spleen work harder and thus wears the spleen out more quickly. If one's spleen is very robust, eating uncooked, raw foods may not be so damaging, but especially for women, their spleens are already weak because of their monthly menses overtaxing the spleen *vis à vis* blood production. It is also a fact of life that the spleen typically becomes weak with age.

More importantly, chilled foods directly damage the spleen. Chilled, frozen foods and drinks neutralize the spleen's yang qi. The process of digestion is the process of turning all foods and drinks to 100°

Fahrenheit soup within the stomach so that it may undergo distillation. If the spleen expends too much yang qi just warming the food up, then it will become damaged and weak. Therefore, all foods and liquids should be eaten and drunk at room temperature at the least and better at body temperature. The more signs and symptoms of spleen vacuity a person presents, such as fatigue, chronically loose stools, undigested food in the stools, cold hands and feet, dizziness on standing up, and aversion to cold, the more closely she should avoid uncooked, chilled foods and drinks.

In addition, sugars and sweets directly damage the spleen. This is because sweet is the flavor which inherently "gathers" in the spleen. It is also an inherently dampening flavor according to Chinese medicine. This means that the body engenders or secretes fluids which gather and collect, transforming into dampness, in response to foods with an excessively sweet flavor. In Chinese medicine, it is said that the spleen is averse to dampness. Dampness is yin and controls or checks yang qi. The spleen's function is based on the transformative and transporting functions of yang qi. Therefore, anything which is excessively dampening can damage the spleen. The sweeter a food is, the more dampening and, therefore, more damaging it is to the spleen.

Another food which is dampening and, therefore, damaging to the spleen is what Chinese doctors call "sodden wheat foods." This means flour products such as bread and noodles. Wheat (as opposed to rice) is damp by nature. When wheat is steamed, yeasted, and/or refined, it becomes even more dampening. In addition, all oils and fats are damp by nature and, hence, may damage the spleen. The more oily or greasy a food is, the worse it is for the spleen. Because milk contains a lot of fat, dairy products are another spleen-damaging, dampness-engendering food. This includes milk, butter, and cheese.

If we put this all together, then ice cream is just about the worst thing a person with a weak, damp spleen could eat. Ice cream is chilled, it is intensely sweet, and it is filled with fat. Therefore, it is a triple whammy when it comes to damaging the spleen. Likewise, pasta smothered in tomato sauce and cheese is a recipe for disaster. Pasta made from wheat flour is dampening, tomatoes are dampening, and cheese is dampening. In addition, what many people don't know is that a glass of fruit juice contains as much sugar as a candy bar, and, therefore, is also very damaging to the spleen and damp-engendering.

As we have seen before, most cases of depression involve an element of liver depression, qi stagnation and stagnant qi leads to stagnation of other substances, such as dampness and phlegm. It is fairly common to encounter a pattern of depression that involves on the one hand a loss of the liver's ability to course and discharge (resulting in a stagnation of qi) and on the other hand a weakening of the spleen's ability to transport and transform (which results in dampness and phlegm). In our clinical experience, a great number of people who experience depression react very favorably to the elimination of both wheat and dairy products from their diet and, in some cases, to the elimination of other gluten-rich grains, such as oats and barley.

Below is a list of specific Western foods which are either uncooked, chilled, too sweet, or too dampening and thus damaging to the spleen. Persons with depression should minimize or avoid these proportional to how weak and damp their spleen is.

Ice cream	Juicy, sweet fruits, such as oranges, peaches, straw-berries, and tomatoes
Sugar	
Candy, especially chocolate	
Milk	Fatty meats
Butter	Fried foods
Cheese	Refined flour products
Margarine	Yeasted bread
Yogurt	Nuts
Raw salads	Alcohol (which is essentially sugar)
Fruit juices	

If the spleen is weak and wet, one should also not eat too much at any one time. A weak spleen can be overwhelmed by a large meal, especially if any of the food is hard to digest. This then results in food stagnation which only impedes the free flow of qi all the more and further damages the spleen.

A clear, bland diet

In Chinese medicine, the best diet for the spleen and, therefore, by extension for most humans, is what is called a "clear, bland diet." This is a diet high in complex carbohydrates such as unrefined grains, especially rice and beans. It is a diet which is high in *lightly cooked* vegetables. It is a diet which is low in fatty meats, oily, greasy, fried foods, and very sweet foods. However, it is not a completely vegetarian diet. Most people, in my experience ,should eat one to two ounces of various types of meat two to four times per week. This animal flesh may be the highly popular but over-touted chicken and fish, but should also include some lean beef, pork, and lamb. Some fresh or cooked fruits may be eaten, but fruit juices should be avoided. In addition, women especially should make an effort to include tofu and tempeh, two soy foods now commonly available in North American grocery stores, in their diet.

If the spleen is weak, then one should eat several smaller meals than one or two large meals. In addition, because rice is 1) neutral in temperature, 2) it fortifies the spleen and supplements the qi, and 3) it eliminates dampness, rice should be the main or staple grain in the diet.

A few problem foods

Coffee

There are a few "problem" foods which deserve special mention. The first of these is coffee. Many people crave coffee for two reasons. First, coffee moves stuck qi. Therefore, if a person suffers from liver depression qi stagnation, temporarily coffee will make them feel like their qi is flowing. Secondly, coffee transforms essence into qi and makes that qi temporarily available to the body. Therefore, people

97

who suffer from spleen and/or kidney vacuity fatigue will get a temporary lift from coffee. They will feel like they have energy. However, once this energy is used up, they are left with a negative deficit. The coffee has transformed some of the essence stored in the kidneys into qi. This qi has been used, and now there is less stored essence. Since the blood and essence share a common source, coffee drinking may ultimately worsen depression associated with blood or kidney vacuities. Tea has a similar effect as coffee in that it transforms yin essence into yang qi and liberates that upward and outward through the body. However, the caffeine in black tea is usually only half as strong as in coffee.

Chocolate

Another problem food is chocolate. Chocolate is a combination of oil, sugar, and cocoa. We have seen that both oil and sugar are dampening and damaging to the spleen. Temporarily, the sugar will boost the spleen qi, but ultimately it will result in "sugar blues" or a hypoglycemic let-down. Cocoa stirs the life gate fire. The life gate fire is another name for kidney yang or kidney fire, and kidney fire is the source of sexual energy and desire. It is said that chocolate is the food of love, and from the Chinese medical point of view, that is true. Since chocolate stimulates kidney fire at the same time as it temporarily boosts the spleen, it does give one a rush of yang qi. In addition, this rush of yang qi does move depression and stagnation, at least short-term. So it makes sense that some people with liver depression, spleen vacuity, and kidney yang debility might crave chocolate.

Alcohol

Alcohol is both damp and hot according to Chinese medical theory. Hence, in English it is referred to as "fire water." It strongly moves the qi and blood. Therefore, persons with liver depression qi stagnation will feel temporarily better from drinking alcohol. However, the sugar in alcohol damages the spleen and engenders dampness which "gums up the works," while the heat (yang) in alcohol can waste the blood (yin) and aggravate or inflame depressive liver heat.

Hot, peppery foods

Spicy, peppery, "hot" foods also move the qi, thereby giving some temporary relief to liver depression qi stagnation. However, like alcohol, the heat in spicy hot foods wastes the blood and can inflame yang.

Sour foods

In Chinese medicine, the sour flavor is inherently astringing and constricting. Therefore, people with liver depression qi stagnation should be careful not to use vinegar and other intensely sour foods. Such sour flavored foods will only aggravate the qi stagnation by astringing and restricting the qi and blood all the more. This is also why sweet and sour foods, such as orange juice and tomatoes are particularly bad for people with liver depression and spleen vacuity. The sour flavor astringes and constricts the qi, while the sweet flavor damages the spleen and engenders dampness.

Diet sodas

In my experience (BF), diet sodas seem to contain something that damages the Chinese idea of the kidneys. They may not damage the spleen the same way that sugared sodas do, but that does not mean they are healthy and safe. I say that diet sodas damage the kidneys since a number of my patients over the years have reported that, when they drink numerous diet sodas, they experience terminal dribbling, urinary incontinence, and low back and knee soreness and weakness. When they stop drinking diet sodas, these symptoms disappear. Taken as a group, in Chinese medicine, these are kidney vacuity symptoms. Since many people aged 40 and above suffering from depression have concomitant kidney vacuity, I typically recommend such patients to steer clear of diet sodas so as not to weaken their kidneys any further or faster.

Foods which help nourish the blood

Qi & Wei

According to Chinese dietary therapy, all foods contain varying proportions of qi and *wei*. Qi means the ability to catalyze or promote yang function, while *wei* (literally meaning flavor) refers to a food's ability to nourish or construct yin substance. Since blood is relatively yin compared to qi being yang, a certain amount of food high in *wei* is necessary for a person to engender and transform blood. Foods which are high in *wei* as compared to qi are those which tend to be heavy, dense, greasy or oily, meaty or bloody. All animal products contain more *wei* than vegetable products. At the same time, black beans or, even better, black soybeans contain more *wei* than celery or lettuce.

When people suffer from depression concomitant with anxiety due to blood vacuity failing to nourish the heart and quiet the spirit or yin vacuity failing to control yang, they usually need to eat slightly more foods high in *wei*. This includes animal proteins and products, such as meat and eggs. It is said that flesh foods are very "compassionate" to the human body. This word recognizes the fact that the animal's life has had to be sacrificed to produce this type of food. It also recognizes that, because such food is so close to the human body itself, it is especially nutritious. Therefore, when people suffer from blood and yin vacuity depression, eating some animal products usually is helpful and sometimes is down right necessary.

Animal foods vs. vegetarianism

Based on my many years of clinical experience (BF), I have seen many Westerners adhering to a strict vegetarian diet develop, after several years, blood or yin vacuity patterns. This is especially the case in women who lose blood every month and must build babies out of the blood and yin essence. When women who are strict vegetarians come to me with various complaints, if they present the signs and symptoms of blood vacuity, such as a fat, pale tongue, pale face, pale nails, and pale lips, heart palpitations, insomnia, and fatigue with a fine, forceless pulse, I typically recommend that they include a little animal food in their diet. In such cases, they commonly report to me how much better they feel immediately—how much more energy they have.

The downside of eating meat—besides the ethical issues—are that foods which are high in *wei* also tend to be harder to digest and to engender phlegm and dampness. Therefore, such foods should only be eaten in very small amounts at any one time. In addition, the weaker the person's spleen or the more phlegm and dampness they already have, the less such foods they should eat.

Remember above we said that the process of digestion first consisted of turning the food and drink ingested into 100° soup in the stomach. Therefore, soups and broths made out of animal flesh are the easiest and most digestible way of adding some animal-quality *wei* to a person's diet. When eating flesh itself, this should probably be limited to only one to two ounces per serving and only three or four such servings per week. According to Chinese dietary theory, the best foods for engendering and transforming blood and yin essence are organ meats and red or dark meats. This includes beef, buffalo, venison, and lamb and dark meat from chicken, turkey, goose, and duck. White meat fish and white meat fowl are less effective for building blood. However, white meat pork is also OK as is ham.

One good recipe for adding more digestible *wei* to the diet of a person who is blood vacuous is to take a marrow bone and boil this with some cut vegetables, especially root vegetables, and black beans or black soybeans. Such a marrow bone, black bean, and vegetable soup is easy to digest and yet rich in *wei*.

The proverbial glass of hot milk

The fact that milk is rich in *wei* is exactly why it is a soporific or sleep-inducer according to Chinese medicine. Being high in *wei* or yin, milk helps control counterflowing, hyperactive yang. In depression cases where liver depression qi stagnation combines with significant yin vacuity, and insomnia is one of the main symptoms, drinking some warm milk before bedtime may actually help the insomnia *as long as the person does not suffer from either dampness or phlegm*. For persons with phlegm heat pattern depression which also presents with insomnia, drinking a warm glass of milk before bed will typically make both their depression and their insomnia worse! This is the beauty of Chinese medicine. It allows one to determine on an individual basis whether any food, medicine, or activity will be good for their particular pattern of imbalance. The Chinese would say that blending a whole egg into boiling milk makes this time-tested remedy even more effective for enriching yin.

The most important thing to remember about diet is that if: A) the spleen is healthy and strong, B) one eats primarily a clear, bland diet with a little bit of animal food, C) one gets sufficient exercise, but D) one does not overtax oneself, then one will manufacture good amounts of qi and blood. Whatever of this qi and blood is left unconsumed at the end of the day will be transformed into acquired essence that night. This is the safest way of engendering and transforming blood and yin via the diet. If one loads up on foods which are high in *wei*, in theory, these may supplement yin and nourish blood. However, if, in fact, they gum up the qi mechanism, the net result will be less qi and blood, not more, and one will have complicated their case even more by creating phlegm and dampness to boot.

In the following chapter, the reader will find some specific recipes combining Chinese herbs and foods for regulating the qi and quieting the spirit to help depression.

Some last words on diet

In conclusion, Western patients are always asking me (BF) what they should eat in order to cure their disease. However, when it comes to diet, sad to say, the issue is not so much what to eat as what not to eat. Diet most definitely plays a major role in the cause and perpetuation of many people's depression, but, except in the case of vegetarians suffering from blood or yin vacuities, the issue is mainly what to avoid or minimize, not what to eat. Most of us know that coffee, chocolate, sugars and sweets, oils and fats, and alcohol are not good for us. Most of us know that we should be eating more complex carbohydrates and freshly cooked vegetables and less fatty meats. However, it's one thing to know these things and another to follow what we know.

To be perfectly honest, a clear bland diet *à la* Chinese medicine is not the most exciting diet in the world. It is the traditional diet of most lower and lower middle class peoples around the world living in temperate climates. It is the traditional diet of most of my readers' great grandparents. The point I am making here is that our modern Western diet which is high in oils and fats, high in sugars and sweets, high in animal proteins, and proportionally high in uncooked, chilled foods and drinks is a relatively recent aberration, and you can't fool Mother Nature.

When one switches to the clear, bland diet of Chinese medicine, at first one may suffer from cravings for more "flavorful" food. These cravings are, in many cases, actually associated with food "allergies." In other words, we may crave what is actually not good for us similar to a drunk's craving alcohol. After a few days, these cravings tend to disappear and we may be amazed that we don't miss some of our convenience or "comfort" foods as much as we thought we would. If one has been addicted to a food like sugar for many years, it does not take much to "fall off the wagon" and be addicted again. Therefore, perseverance is the key to long-term success. As the Chinese say, a million is made up of nothing but lots of ones, and a bucket is quickly filled by steady drips and drops.

Exercise

Exercise is the second of what we call the three free therapies. According to Chinese medicine, regular and adequate exercise has two basic benefits. First, exercise promotes the movement of the qi and quickening of the blood. Since almost all depression involves liver depression qi stagnation, it is obvious that exercise is an important therapy for coursing the liver and rectifying the qi. Secondly, exercise benefits the spleen. The spleen's movement and transportation of the digestate is dependent upon the qi mechanism. The qi mechanism describes the function of the qi in upbearing the pure and downbearing the turbid parts of digestion. For the qi mechanism to function properly, the qi must be flowing normally and freely. Since exercise moves and rectifies the qi, it also helps regulate and rectify the qi mechanism. This then results in the spleen's movement and transportation of foods and liquids and its subsequent engendering and transforming of the qi and blood. Because spleen qi vacuity and dampness accumulation typically complicate most people's depression and because a healthy spleen checks and controls a depressed liver, exercise treats one of the other commonly encountered disease mechanisms in the majority of Westerner's suffering from depression. Therefore, it is easy to see that regular, adequate exercise is a vitally important component of any person's regime for either preventing or treating depression.

What kind of exercise is best for depression?

Aerobics

In my experience, I (BF) find aerobic exercise to be the most beneficial for most people with depression. By aerobic exercise, I mean *any physical activity which raises one's heartbeat 80% above their normal resting rate and keeps it there for at least 20 minutes.* To calculate your normal resting heart rate, place your fingers over the pulsing artery on the front side of your neck. Count the beats for 15 seconds and then multiply by four. This gives you your beats per minute or BPM. Now multiply your BPM by 0.8. Take the resulting number and add it to your resting BPM. This gives you your aerobic threshold of BPM. Next engage in any physical activity you like. After you have been exercising for five minutes, take your pulse for 15 seconds once again at the artery on the front side of your throat. Again multiply the resulting count by four and this tells you your current BPM. If this number is less than your aerobic threshold BPM, then you know you need to exercise harder or faster. Once you get your heart rate up to your aerobic threshold, then you need to keep exercising at the same level of intensity for at least 20 minutes. In order to insure that one is keeping their heartbeat high enough for long enough, one should recount their pulse every five minutes or so.

Depending on one's age and physical condition, different people will have to exercise harder to reach their aerobic threshold than others. For some, simply walking briskly will raise their heartbeat 80% above their resting rate. For others, they will need to do calisthenics, running, swimming, racket ball, or some other, more strenuous exercise. It really does not matter what the exercise is as long as it raises your heartbeat 80% above your resting rate and keeps it there for 20 minutes. However, there are two other criteria that should be met. One, the exercise should be something that is not too boring. If it is too boring, then you may have a hard time keeping up your schedule. Since most people do find aerobic exercises such as running, stationary bicycles, and stair-steppers boring, it is good to listen to music or watch TV in order to distract your mind from the tedium. Secondly, the type of exercise should not cause any damage to any parts of the body. For instance, running on pavement may cause knee problems for some people. Therefore, you should pick a type of exercise you enjoy but also one which will not cause any problems.

When doing aerobic exercise, it is best to exercise either every day or every other day. If one does not do their aerobics at least once every 72 hours, then its cumulative effects will not be as great. Therefore, I recommend my patients with depression do some sort of aerobic exercises every day or every other day, three to four times per week *at least*. The good news is that there is no real need to exercise more than 30 minutes at any one time. Forty-five minutes per session is not going to be all that much better than 25 minutes per session. And 25 minutes four times per week is very much better than one hour once a week.

Weight lifting

Recent research has also demonstrated that weight lifting can help relieve depression in women of all ages.[17] Therefore, lifting weights is recommendable on the days when one is not doing aerobics. In that case, one can do aerobics three to four days a week and lift weights the other three days. In general, one should not lift weights every day unless one varies the muscle groups they are working each day. In the study on weight lifting and depression cited above, the women lifted weights which were 45-87% as heavy as the maximum they could lift at one time. Those women who lifted weights closer to the top end of this range saw the greatest benefits. These women lifted weights three days per week for 10 weeks, gradually increasing the amount of weight they lifted at each session.

Because weight lifting requires some initial training and education in order to do safely and properly, it is recommended taking a few classes either at a local YMCA or recreation center or from a private trainer. When aerobics are alternated with weight lifting, one has a really comprehensive training regime designed to benefit both one's cardiovascular system and one's muscles, tendons, ligaments, and bones. In addition, regular weight-bearing exercise is also important for preventing osteoporosis.

Too much exercise

While the vast majority of people with depression will benefit from more exercise, there are a few who actually need less physical activity. As we have seen, all stirring or activity entails a consumption of yin by yang. If a person is either constitutionally yin vacuous or, due to some circumstance, like aging, enduring disease, extreme blood loss, excessive births, or lactation, has become yin vacuous, then too much exercise or physical activity can worsen that yin vacuity. This is mostly seen in women with thin bodily

---

[17] "Depression and Weight Training", *Harvard Women's Health Watch*, Vol. IV, #6, February 1997, reporting on research published in the *Journal of Gerontology*, January 1997

constitutions who overexercise, such as professional athletes, or in women who suffer from anorexia and bulimia.

Body fat in Chinese medicine is nothing other than yin. Therefore, people who are very thinly built tend to have less yin to begin with. If, through exercise, one reduces their body fat even more, it may become so insufficient that yin can no longer control yang. In women, such an insufficiency of yin blood due to overconsumption in turn due to too much exercise usually manifests itself first as cessation of menstruation or amenorrhea. However, it is also possible for drug use, especially types of "speed", or anorexia and bulimia to also result in an overconsumption of yin leading to amenorrhea on the one hand and increased mental agitation and insomnia on the other. Here I am using the term bulimia as binging and purging, *i.e.*, eating but vomiting back up whatever has been ingested. Although the woman may be eating, often she still is not getting sufficient yin nourishment. It is also not uncommon to find an attraction to speed, a tendency to over exercise, and a tendency to anorexia all in the same woman.

In such women, it may be necessary to actually curtail the amount of exercise they are getting. One knows if the amount of exercise they are getting is a good amount if they feel refreshed and invigorated a couple of hours after the exercise is over. If, on the other hand, one feels even more fatigued or feels even more nervous and jittery, or if exercise during the day leads to night sweats and insomnia at night, then one should consider actually doing less exercise.

Deep relaxation

As we have seen above, depression is commonly associated with liver depression qi stagnation. If liver depression endures or is severe, it typically transforms into heat or fire. Heat or fire being yang, consume and exhaust yin and blood. Thus yang qi moves frenetically upward, disturbing the heart spirit, causing anxiety and agitation at the same time as depression. Therefore, liver depression qi stagnation is often at the root of depression. In Chinese medicine, liver depression comes from not fulfilling all one's desires. But as we have also seen above, no adult can fulfill all their desires. This is why a certain amount of liver depression is endemic among adults. When our desires are frustrated, our qi becomes depressed. This then creates emotional depression and easy anger or irritability. In Chinese medicine, anger is nothing other than the venting of pent up qi in the liver. When qi becomes depressed in the liver, it accumulates like hot air in a balloon. Eventually, that hot, depressed, angry qi has to go somewhere. So when there is a little more frustration or stress, then this angry qi in the liver vents itself as irritability, anger, shouting, or nasty words, and it moves upward in the body to disturb the spirit in the heart. In Chinese medicine, it is a basic statement of fact that, "Anger results in the qi ascending."

Essentially, this type of anger and irritability are due to a maladaptive coping response that is typically learned at a young age. When we feel frustrated or stressed, stymied by or angry about something, most of us tense our muscles and especially the muscles in our upper back and shoulders, neck, and jaws. At the same time, many of us will hold our breath. In Chinese medicine, the sinews are governed by the liver. This tensing of the muscles, *i.e.*, the sinews, constricts the flow of qi in the channels and network vessels. Since it is the liver which is responsible for the coursing and discharging of this qi, such tensing of the sinews leads to liver depression qi stagnation. Because the lungs govern the downward spreading and movement of the qi, holding our breath due to stress or frustration only worsens this tendency of the qi not to move and, therefore, to become depressed in the Chinese medical idea of the liver.

Therefore, deep relaxation is the third of the three free therapies. For deep relaxation to be therapeutic medically, it needs to be more than just mental equilibrium. It needs to be somatic or bodily relaxation as well as mental repose. Most of us no longer recognize that every thought we think and feeling we feel is actually a felt physical sensation somewhere in our body. The words we use to describe emotions are all abstract nouns, such as anger, depression, sadness, and melancholy. However, in Chinese medicine, *every emotion is associated with a change in the direction or flow of qi.* As we have said above, anger makes the qi move upward. Fear, on the other hand, makes the qi move downward. Therefore, anger "makes our gorge rise" or "blow our top", while fear may cause a "sinking feeling" or make us "pee in our pants." These colloquial expressions are all based on the age-old wisdom that all thoughts and emotions are not just mental but also bodily events. This is why it is not just enough to clear one's mind. Clearing one's mind is good, but for really marked therapeutic results, it is even better if one clears one's mind at the same time as relaxing every muscle in the body as well as the breath.

Guided deep relaxation tapes

A very efficient and effective way to practice such mental and physical deep relaxation is to do a daily, guided, progressive, deep relaxation audiotape. Guided meaning that a narrator on the tape leads one through the process of deep relaxation. Such tapes are progressive since they lead one through the body in a progressive manner, first relaxing one body part and then moving on to another. For instance, the narrator may say something to the effect that, as you exhale, you should feel your forehead get heavy and relaxed, softening and expanding, becoming warm and heavy. As you exhale again, now feel your cheeks get heavy and relaxed, softening and expanding, becoming warm and heavy. Breathe in and breathe out, letting your breath go without hindrance or hesitation. Breathing out, now feel your jaw muscles become heavy and relaxed, expanding and softening, becoming warm and heavy, etc., etc. throughout the entire body until one comes to the bottoms of one's feet.

There are innumerable such tapes on the market. These are usually sold in health food stores, New Age music and supply stores, or in bookstores with a good selection of New Age books. Over the years of suggesting this method of deep relaxation to my patients, I have found that each patient will have her own preferences in terms of the type of voice, male or female, the choice of words and imagery, whether there is background music or not, and the actual pace of the progression through the body, some narrators speaking a slightly different rate and rhythm. Therefore, I suggest listening to and even purchasing more than one such tape. One should find a tape which they like and can listen to without internal criticism or comment, going along like a cloud in the sky as the narrator's voice blows away all your mental and bodily stress and tension. If one has more than one tape, one can also switch every now and again from tape to tape so as not to become bored with the process or desensitized to the instructions.

Key things to look for in a good relaxation tape

In order to get the full therapeutic effect of such deep relaxation tapes, there are several key things to check for. First, be sure that the tape is a guided tape and not a subliminal relaxation tape. Subliminal tapes usually have music and any instructions to relax are given so quietly that they are not consciously heard. Although such tapes can help you feel relaxed when you do them, ultimately they do not teach you how to relax as a skill which can be consciously practiced and refined. Secondly, make sure the tape starts from the top of the body and works downward. Remember, anger makes the qi go upward in the body, and people with irritability and easy anger due to liver depression qi stagnation already have too much qi rising upward in their bodies. Such depressed qi typically needs not only to be moved but also downborne. Third, make sure the tape instructs you to relax your physical body. If you do not relax all your muscles or sinews, the qi cannot flow freely and the liver cannot be coursed. Depression is not resolved, and there will not be the same medically therapeutic effect. And lastly, be sure the tape instructs you to let your breath go with each exhalation. One of the symptoms of liver depression is a stuffy feeling in the chest which we then unconsciously try to relieve by sighing. Letting each exhalation go completely helps the lungs push

110

the qi downward. This allows the lungs to control the liver at the same time as it downbears upwardly counterflowing angry liver qi.

The importance of daily practice

I (BF) was once taken on a field trip to a hospital clinic where they were using deep relaxation as a therapy with patients with high blood pressure, heart disease, stroke, migraines, and insomnia. The doctors at this clinic showed us various graphs plotting their research data on how such daily, progressive deep relaxation can regulate the blood pressure and body temperature and improve the appetite, digestion, elimination, sleep, energy, and mood. One of the things they said has stuck with me for 15 years: "Small results in 100 days, big results in 1,000." This means that if one does such daily, progressive deep relaxation *every single day for 100 days*, one will definitely experience certain results. What are these "small" results? These small results are improvements in all the parameters listed above: blood pressure, body temperature, appetite, digestion, elimination, sleep, energy, and mood. If these are "small" results, then what are the "big" results experienced in 1,000 days of practice? The "big" results are a change in how one reacts to stress—in other words, a change in one's very personality or character.

What these doctors in Shanghai stressed and what I have also experienced both personally and with my patients: the effects of this relaxation are cumulative, meaning that the longer one can practice this routine on a consistent daily basis the greater and more lasting the effects will be.

It is vitally important to do such daily, guided, progressive deep relaxation every single day, day in and day out for a solid three months at least and for a continuous three years at best. If one does such progressive, somatic deep relaxation every day, *one will see every parameter or measurement of health and well-being improve.* If one does this kind of deep relaxation only sporadically, missing a day here and there, it will feel good when you do it, but it will not have the marked, cumulative therapeutic effects it can. Therefore,

111

perseverance is the real key to getting the benefits of deep relaxation.

The real test

Doing such a daily deep relaxation regime is like hitting tennis balls against a wall or hitting a bucket of balls at a driving range. It is only practice; it is not the real game itself. Doing a daily deep relaxation regime is not only in order to relieve one's immediate stress and strain. It is to learn a new skill, a new way to react to stress. The ultimate goal is to learn how to breathe out and immediately relax all one's muscles in the body in reaction to stress, rather than the common but unhealthy maladaptation to stress of holding one's breath and tensing one's muscles. By doing such deep relaxation day after day, one learns how to relax any and every muscle in the body quickly and efficiently. Then, as soon as one recognizes they are feeling frustrated, stressed out, or uptight, they can immediately remedy those feelings at the same time as coursing their liver and rectifying their qi. This is the real test, the game of life. "Small results in 100 days, big results in 1,000."

Simple Home Remedies for Depression

Although faulty diet, lack of adequate exercise, and too much stress are the most significant contributing factors to depression according to Chinese medicine and, therefore, diet, exercise, and deep relaxation are the most important parts of every person's treatment and prevention of depression, there are a number of simple Chinese home remedies to help relieve the symptoms of depression.

Chinese aromatherapy

In Chinese medicine, the qi is seen as a type of wind or vapor. The Chinese character for qi shows wind blowing over a rice field. In addition, smells are often referred to as a thing's qi. Therefore, there is a close relationship between smells carried through the air and the flow of qi in a person's body. Although aromatherapy has not been a major part of professionally practiced Chinese medicine for almost a thousand years, there is a simple aromatherapy treatment which one can do at home which can help alleviate irritability, depression, nervousness, anxiety, and insomnia.

In Chinese, *Chen Xiang* means "sinking fragrance." It is the name of Lignum Aquilariae Agallochae or Eaglewood. This is a frequent ingredient in Asian incense formulas. In Chinese medicine, Aquilaria is classified as a qi-rectifying medicinal. When used as a boiled decoction or "tea", Aquilaria moves the qi and stops pain, downbears upward counterflow and regulates the middle (*i.e.*, the spleen and stomach), and promotes the kidneys' grasping of the qi sent down by the lungs. I believe that the word sinking in this herb's name refers to this medicinal's downbearing of upwardly counterflowing qi. Such upwardly counterflowing eventually must accumulate in the heart, disturbing and causing restlessness of the heart spirit. When this medicinal wood is burnt and its smoke is inhaled as a medicinal incense, its downbearing and spirit-calming function is emphasized.

One can buy Aquilaria or *Chen Xiang* from Chinese herb stores in Chinatowns, Japantowns, or Koreatowns in major urban areas. One can also buy it from Chinese medical practitioners who have their own pharmacies. (See below for addresses, phone numbers, and fax numbers for companies selling Chinese herbs by mail.) It is best to use the powdered variety. However, powder may be made by putting a small piece of this aromatic wood in a coffee grinder. It is also ok to use small bits of the wood if powder is not available. Next one needs to buy a roll of incense charcoals. Place one charcoal in non-flammable dish and light it with a match. Then sprinkle a few pinches of Aquilaria powder on the lit charcoal. As the smoke rises, breathe in deeply. This can be done on a regular basis one or more times per day or on an as-needed basis by those suffering from restlessness, nervousness, anxiety, and irritability. For those who are experiencing depression, one can do this "treatment" on a regular basis at least three times per week.

This Chinese aromatherapy with Lignum Aquilariae Agallochae is very cheap and effective. We know of no side effects or contraindications.

Magnet therapy

The Chinese have used magnet therapy since at least the Tang dynasty (618-907 CE). Placing magnets on the body is a safe and painless way of stimulating acupuncture points without inserting needles through the skin. Since magnets can be taped onto points and "worn" for days at a time, Chinese magnet therapy is able to provide easy, low cost, continuous treatment. It is also possible to tape on magnets at night and to wear them to bed. Special adhesive magnets for stimulating acupuncture points, such as Accu-Band Magnets, Corimag, or Epaule Patch TDK Magnets, may be purchased from:

Oriental Medical Supply Co.
1950 Washington St.
Braintree, MA 02184
Tel: (617) 331-3370 or 800-323-1839 Fax: (617) 335-5779

These magnets range in strength from 400-9,000 gauss, the unit measuring magnetic strength. For the treatments below, one can try 400-800 gauss magnets.

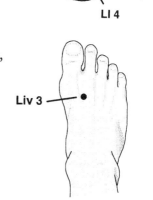

LI 4

Liv 3

There is a set of four points which we mentioned earlier called the Four Gates. The Four Gates are comprised by two points. The first point, *He Gu* (LI 4), is located on the top of the hand, between the thumb and the index finger, at the highest spot of the muscle when the thumb and index finger are brought close together. The second point, *Tai Chong* (Liv 3) is located on the top of the foot, between the first and second toes, about two inches away from the margin of the web towards the body.

These points regulate the upbearing of the clear and downbearing of the turbid, calm the mind and settle the spirit. It isn't always necessary to treat all Four Gates and for some people the sedative effect is too great if it's done this way. One can reach dramatic results by treating these points contra laterally, meaning, one point is done on the right side while the other is done on the left. To treat the Four Gates with magnets, one can tape a magnet with the south

115

side down on *Tai Chong*, and a magnet with its north side down on *He Gu*.

For women, the hand point (*He Gu*) should be on the right side and the foot point (*Tai Chong*) on the left, while for men, the hand point should be on the left and the foot point on the right. According to Chinese medicine left and right are a yin-yang pair. The left corresponds to yang which is associated with the male element. The right corresponds to yin and the female element.

Tai Chong can be combined in the same fashion with another very helpful point, *Nei Guan* (Per 6). This point is located on the inner side of the forearm between the two tendons. When used in combination, *Tai Chong* and *Nei Guan* rectifies the qi and resolves depression, loosens the chest and quiets the spirit. These two points are also best treated with magnets applied contra laterally according to the same principle for choosing left and right described above.

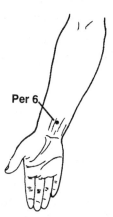

For any of these two point combinations, apply the magnets during the day and leave in place for four to six hours. Then remove them. If good results have been achieved, repeat this the next day for the same length of time. Do not use these point combinations during sleep or late at night.

When insomnia is the main feature in depression, magnets can also be used. It is said in Chinese medicine that the ability to open and close the eyes has to do with the yang qi in two specific channels. These channels are called the *yin qiao mai* and the *yang qiao mai*. This translates as the yin and yang springing vessels. These two vessels both begin on the feet and meet at the eyes. The *yang qiao mai* carries yang qi upward to the head and specifically to the eyes. When this vessel is full of yang qi, the eyes are open and the person is awake. When this yang qi moves from the *yang qiao mai* into the

116

yin qiao mai and is thence led back down into the lower and interior parts of the body, then the eyes close and one can go to sleep. Therefore, the yin and yang in the body that govern sleep and wake can be regulated by balancing the yin and yang qi in these two special vessels.

In most types of insomnia, yang qi is too full and is counterflowing upward out of control. In order to promote sleep, yin must be nourished in order to "magnetize" or attract yang to move back downward and inward. In insomnia, the yang qi in the *yang qiao mai* is too full or replete, while the yin qi in the *yin qiao mai* is vacuous and insufficient. In order to re-establish the balance between yin and yang in these two vessels, one needs to drain the *yang qiao mai* and supplement the *yin qiao mai*. In acupuncture, this can be done by using gold needles to supplement the meeting point of the *yin qiao mai* and silver needles to drain the *yang qiao mai*. It is also possible to drain these points with copper and zinc needles respectively. However, this requires puncturing the skin and should only be done by a professional acupuncturist.

Happily, one can get the same effect by taping small magnets over these points. The meeting or command point of the *yin qiao mai* is called *Zhao Hai* (Ki 6). It is located one inch beneath the tip of the inner anklebone in a small depression below that bone. The meeting point of the *yang qiao mai* is called *Shen Mai* (Bl 62). It is located one inch below the tip of the outer anklebone, also in a small depression. In order to drain the yang qi from *Shen Mai*, tape a small body magnet south side down over this point just before bed at night. In order to supplement the yin qi at *Zhao Hai*, tape a small body magnet north side down over that point just before bed at night. Do this to both sets of points on both feet. Leave these magnets in place overnight, and remove them each morning when you wake. This can be done night after night until one is able to sleep without their aid.

Chinese self-massage

Massage, including self-massage, is a highly developed part of traditional Chinese medicine. The self-massage regime below is specifically designed as a home remedy for depression. For more Chinese self-massage regimes, the readers should see Fan Ya-li's *Chinese Self-massage Therapy: The Easy Way to Health* also published by Blue Poppy Press.

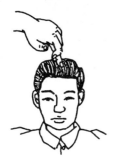

Begin by pressing and kneading the very center and top of the skull. This is acupoint *Bai Hui* (GV 20). It is the most yang point in the body and is the meeting place of all the yang channels and vessels. It is especially useful for calming the spirit, soothing the liver, and subduing hyperactive yang. Do this approximately 100 times.

Next, knead with the fingertips of both hands the acupoint located at the inner ends of the eyebrows. This area corresponds to the point *Zhan Zhu* (Bl 2). It is the place where the yang qi traveling up the *yang qiao mai* connects with the *yin qiao mai* which leads downward. Knead this area approximately 30 times.

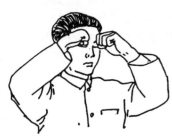

Third, with the index fingers and thumbs, wipe the upper edge of the eye bone and then the lower edge. Work from the inner corners of the eyes to the outer corners. This helps move the yang qi in the eyes downward and keeps it from congesting in the *yang qiao mai* in the eyes. Do this 20-30 times.

Fourth, rub the palms of the hands vigorously together until they feel warm. Then place these warm palms over both eyes. Cover the eyes thus for 30-60 seconds and then lightly rub the closed eyes approximately 10 times.

Fifth, press and knead the acupoint *Feng Chi* (GB 20) with the thumbs. This point is located in the depression between the mastoid process, the bone behind the ear, and the strap muscles which connect at the base of the skull. The point is located approximately one inch within the hairline on most people. It is a point most people instinctively massage when they have a tension head or stiff neck. Do this 30-50 times, massaging both points with both hands at the same time.

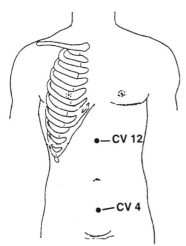

Sixth, rub circles around the center of the upper and the lower abdomen. The point in the middle of the upper abdomen is called *Zhong Wan* (CV 12). The point in the center of the lower abdomen is called *Guan Yuan* (CV 4). Rub these first clockwise and then counterclockwise approximately 100 times each point in each direction.

119

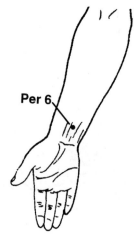

Seventh, press and knead the acupoint *Nei Guan* (Per 6). This point is located on the inner side of the forearm in between the two tendons. It is located approximately 1.5 inches upward from the wrist. First press and knead with the thumb of one hand, and then press and knead with the thumb of the other. Do this approximately 30-50 times on each side. This point helps soothe the liver, regulate the qi, and quiet the spirit.

Eighth, press and knead the point *Shen Men* (Ht 7). This is located on the inner side of the forearm at the crease of the wrist right below the base of the little or "pinky" finger. Massage the points on both wrists 30-50 times each. This point clears heat from the heart and quiets the spirit.

Now, press and knead the point *He Gu* (LI 4). This point is located on the top of the hand, between the thumb and the index finger; at the highest spot of the muscle when the thumb and index finger are brought close together. Choose the hand on one side and then move contra laterally to the opposite foot. Here on the foot press and knead *Tai Chong* (Liv 3) located on the top of the foot between the first and second toes, about two inches

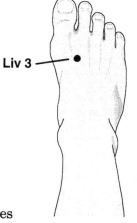

away from the margin of the web towards the body. Do *Tai Chong* on the other foot and then move to do *He Gu* on the other hand. This will help open the Four Gates as seen on the section on magnet therapy above.

Then knead and press *Zu San Li* (St 36). This point is located three inches below the lower, outside edge of the kneecap when the leg is bent. It is located in a depression between the muscles of the lower leg. Massage this point 30-50 times on each side. This point regulates the qi and leads upwardly counterflowing yang qi downward.

Follow this by pressing and kneading *San Yin Jiao* (Sp 6). This point is located three inches above the tip of the inner ankle bone on the back side of the lower leg bone. It is the meeting place of the liver, spleen, and kidney channels. It is very effective for stimulating the production of yin blood in the body which can then "magnetize" yang qi back downward.

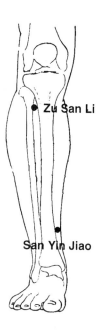

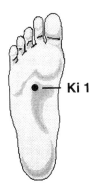

And lastly, rub the depression just behind and to the side of the ball of the foot. This point is called *Yong Quan* (Ki 1). If *Bai Hui* (GV 20) is the most yang point in the body, *Yong Quan* is the most yin.

Stimulating this point helps to lead counterflowing yang qi back downward to its lower source. Rub this point with the palm of the opposite hand until it feels hot. Repeat this on the other foot.

This self-massage regime should take between 20 minutes and one half hour. It should be done every evening just before bed. When doing each massage manipulation, you should try to calmly focus on the physical sensations under your hands and not let your mind wander to your day's worries and affairs.

121

Seven star hammering

A seven star hammer is a small hammer or mallet with seven small needles embedded in its head. Nowadays in China, it is often called a skin or dermal needle. It is one of the ways a person can stimulate various acupuncture points without actually inserting a needle into the body. Seven star hammers can be used either for people who are afraid of regular acupuncture, for children, or for those who wish to treat their condition at home. When the points to be stimulated are on the front of the body, this technique can be done by oneself. When they are located on the back of the body, this technique can be done by a family member or friend. This is a very easy technique which does not require any special training or expertise.

At least part of the seven star treatment for depression will require a helper. First, disinfect all the areas of the skin which are going to be tapped. Then begin by lightly tapping on the back of the neck. One should lightly tap all along the center of the spine on the neck as well as up and down the strap muscles to either side of the spinal column. Then one should lightly tap acupoints *Feng Chi* (GB 20). The location of these points behind the mastoid processes behind the ears has been described in the section on Chinese self-massage above (see page 119). If one suffers from depressive heat with red eyes, red face, headache, and/or dizziness, one can tap till the points bleed just a little bit. This helps drain heat or fire from the upper body. Otherwise tap until the skin is simply flushed red.

Next, tap all over the sacrum lightly until it turns a light red color.

Then tap the center of the sternum lightly; there is a point in the midline of the sternum, midway between the two nipples. This point, *Shan Zhong* (Ren 17) opens up the chest, relieves anxiety, irritability and has a calming but invigorating effect. Proceed to the sides of the body, tap the area on the midaxillary line, in the space between the 5 and 6 ribs (the nipples are between the 4 and 5 ribs); this area corresponds to the point *Da Bao* (Sp 21) which opens up the chest, relaxes the diaphragm and helps circulate stagnant qi in the whole thoracic region.

Follow this by tapping *Nei Guan* (Per 6), *Shen Men* (Ht 7), and *San Yin Jiao* (Sp 6) in that order. Then tap *He Gu* (LI 4) and *Tai Chong* (Liv 3) contra laterally. The locations of these five points have also been given under the section on Chinese self-massage above (see pages 120-121).

If there is headache due to ascendant hyperactivity of liver yang, tap over both temples. If the headache is severe, tap till just a little blood is let.

If there is any bleeding, wipe the area with a cotton swab moistened in alcohol or hydrogen peroxide. Then take a dry cotton ball and press the area. Between treatments, soak the seven star hammer in alcohol or hydrogen peroxide and do not share hammers between people in order to prevent any infection from one person to another. Seven star hammers are very cheap. So each person can easily afford to have their own. They can also be purchased from Oriental Medical Supply Co. whose address and phone numbers are given in the section on Chinese magnet therapy above.

Thread moxibustion

Thread moxibustion refers to burning extremely tiny cones or "threads" of aged Oriental mugwort directly on top of certain acupuncture points. When done correctly, this is a very simple and effective way of adding yang qi to the body without causing a burn or scar. Since most people with depression suffer from at least an element of spleen qi and possible kidney yang vacuity, adding yang qi to the body is a good idea in many people with depression. However, if you suffer from depressive heat or yin vacuity, you should probably consult a professional practitioner before using this self-treatment.

To do thread moxa, one must first purchase the finest grade Japanese moxa wool. This is available from Oriental Medical Supply Co. mentioned above under magnet therapy. It is listed under the name Gold Direct Moxa. Pinch off a very small amount of this loose moxa wool and roll it lightly between the thumb and forefinger. What you want to wind up with is a very loose, very thin thread of moxa smaller than a grain of rice. It is important that this thread not be too large or too tightly wrapped.

Next, rub a very thin film of Tiger Balm or Temple of Heaven Balm on the point to be moxaed. These are camphored Chinese medical salves which are widely available in North American health food stores or from Mayway Corp. whose address, telephone numbers, and fax numbers are given below. Be sure to apply nothing more than the thinnest film of salve. If such a Chinese medicated salve is not available, then wipe the point with a tiny amount of vegetable oil. Stand the thread of moxa up perpendicularly directly over the point to be moxaed. The oil or balm should provide enough stickiness to make the thread stand on end. Light the tread with a burning incense stick. As the thread burns down towards the skin, you will feel more and more heat. Immediately remove the burning thread when you begin to feel the burning thread go from hot to too hot. *Do not burn yourself.* It is better to pull the thread off too soon than too late. In this case, more is not better than enough. (If you do burn yourself, apply some *Ching Wan Hong* ointment. This is a Chinese burn salve which is available at Chinese apothecaries and from Mayway Corp. It is truly wonderful for treating all sorts of burns. It should be in every home's medicine cabinet.)

Having removed the burning thread and extinguished it between your two fingers, repeat this process again. To make this process go faster and more efficiently, one can roll a number of threads before starting the treatment. Each time the thread burns down close to the skin, pinch it off the skin and extinguish it *before* it starts to burn you. If you do this correctly, your skin will get red and hot to the touch but you will not raise a blister. Because everyone's skin is different, the first time you do this, only start out with three or four

124

threads. Each day, increase this number until you reach nine to twelve threads per treatment.

This treatment is especially effective for people in their late 30s and throughout their 40s whose spleen and kidney yang qi has already become weak and insufficient or in older patients of both sexes. Since this treatment actually adds yang qi to the body, this type of thread moxa fortifies the spleen and invigorates the kidneys, warming yang and boosting the qi. Because the stimuli is not that strong at any given treatment, it must be done every day for a number of days. For women who suffer from PMS with pronounced premenstrual fatigue, loose stools, cold hands and feet, low or no libido, and low back or knee pain accompanied by frequent nighttime urination which tends to be copious and clear, we recommend beginning this moxibustion just before ovulation, around day 10 in the cycle. It should then be repeated every day up through day one of the period and then suspended. It can be done for several months in a row, but should not usually be done continuously throughout the year, day in and day out.

There are three points which should be moxaed using this supplementing technique. These are:

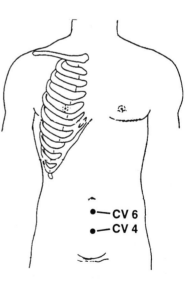

Qi Hai (Conception Vessel 6)

Guan Yuan (Conception Vessel 4)

Zu San Li (Stomach 36)

Qi Hai is located on the midline of the body, two finger widths below the navel. *Guan Yuan* is also located on the midline of the lower abdomen, four finger widths below the navel.

125

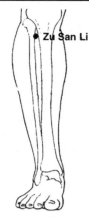

Zu San Li is located four finger widths below the lower edge of the kneecap between the tibia and fibula on the outside edge of the lower leg. However, we *highly* recommend visiting a local professional acupuncturist so that they can teach you how to do this technique safely and effectively and to show you how to locate these three points accurately.

In Chinese medicine, this technique is considered a longevity and health preservation technique. It is great for those people whose yang qi has already begun to decline due to the inevitable aging process. It should not be done by people with ascension of hyperactive liver yang, liver fire, or depressive liver heat. It should also always be done starting from the topmost point and moving downward. This is to prevent leading heat to counterflow upward. If there is any doubt about whether this technique is appropriate for you, please see a professional practitioner for a diagnosis and individualized recommendation.

Chinese medicinal wines

Chinese medicinal wines are part of Chinese dietary therapy. They make use of alcohol's special characteristics as well as a few Chinese herbs or medicinals. Although alcohol is hot and can inflame yang heat, especially liver heat, alcohol moves depressed qi and static blood. It also speeds and increases the medicinal effects of herbs into and in the body. Therefore, one can *cautiously* make and take a number of simple Chinese medicinal wines for various aspects and patterns of depression.

For liver depression with chest oppression, irritability, and insomnia, one can soak 50g each of Flos Albizziae Julibrissinis (*He Huan Pi*), Flos Rosae Rugosae (*Mei Gui Hua*), and Caulis Polygoni Multiflori (*Ye Jiao Teng*) in one quart or fifth of either brandy or

126

vodka for one month. Remove the dregs and drink 1-2 ounces before or after dinner.

For liver depression with chest oppression, rib-side distention and pain, epigastric aching and pain, or breast distention and pain, soak 120g of Rhizoma Cyperi Rotundi (*Xiang Fu*) in one quart or fifth of vodka or brandy for one month, remove the dregs, and take a half ounce or less repeatedly throughout the day. Do not use this formula if there are signs of heat such as red eyes, red face, actual anger, and a red tongue with yellow fur.

For liver depression causing dizziness, headache, or one-sided headache, soak 200g of Fructus Viticis (*Man Jing Zi*) in one quart or fifth of brandy or vodka for one month. Remove the dregs and drink one ounce or so at the time of the dizziness or headache. A slightly more elaborate formula for the same condition consists of 60g of Fructus Viticis (*Man Jing Zi*) and 30g each of Flos Chrysanthemi Morifolii (*Ju Hua*), Radix Ligustici Wallichii (*Chuan Xiong*), Radix Ledebouriellae Divaricatae (*Fang Feng*), and Herba Menthae Haplocalycis (*Bo He*). Make and take the same way as the preceding "wine." This second formula can be cautiously tried even if there are signs and symptoms of depressive heat.

For depressive liver heat with red eyes, headache, and dizziness, soak 125g of Flos Chrysanthemi Morifolii (*Ju Hua*) in one quart of brandy or vodka for one month. Remove the dregs and drink one ounce before or after dinner.

For heart blood-spleen qi vacuity depression, one can try either of two self-made Chinese medicinal wines. The first is made by placing 150g of white Ginseng (Radix Panacis Ginseng, *Ren Shen*) in one quart or fifth of brandy for 1-2 months. Then remove the dregs, and take 1-2 ounces before or after dinner. However, do not use this wine if you display the signs and symptoms of depressive liver heat affecting the head and face. One can also use 150g of Arillus Euphoriae Longanae (*Long Yan Rou*) steeped in one quart or fifth of sake. In that case, drink 1-2 ounces before or after dinner each evening. Do not take this latter wine if you suffer from constipation.

For depression due to phlegm blocking or confounding the portals of the heart, take 120g of Rhizoma Acori Graminei (*Shi Chang Pu*) and soak this in one quart or fifth of vodka for 3-5 days. Then take 10-20ml of the resulting medicinal wine three times per day on an empty stomach.

These are only a few of the Chinese medicinal wines and elixirs that can be made and used at home for the treatment of depression. For more information on Chinese medicinal wines, the reader may see my (BF) *Chinese Medical Wines & Elixirs* also published by Blue Poppy Press.

Chinese medicinal porridges

Like the Chinese medicinal wines discussed above, Chinese medicinal porridges are a specialized part of Chinese dietary therapy. Because porridges are already in the form of 100° soup, they are a particularly good way of eating otherwise nutritious but nevertheless hard-to-digest grains. When Chinese medicinals are cooked along with those grains, one has a high-powered but easily assimilable "health food" of the first order.

For liver depression, qi stagnation pattern of depression, cook 50g of white rice with 10g of Pericarpium Citri Reticulatae Viride (*Qing Pi*). Eat this one time per day. Another possibility is to cook 5g of Flos Pruni (*i.e.*, plum flowers) with 100g of white rice with enough water to make a thin porridge or gruel.

For spleen qi vacuity with pronounced fatigue, cook 30g of Radix Astragali Membranacei (*Huang Qi*) with 6g of Pericarpium Citri Reticulatae (*Chen Pi*) in 600ml of water for 20 minutes. Remove the dregs and then use the resulting medicinal "tea" to cook 50g of white rice. Another possibility for treating spleen qi vacuity fatigue and lack of strength is to take 3g of powdered Radix Panacis Ginseng

(*Ren Shen*) and cook this with 100g of white rice in water. Yet another option is to take 5g of ginseng and 20g of powdered Sclerotium Poriae Cocos (*Fu Ling*) and cook this with 60g of white rice in water. During the last 5-7 minutes of cooking, add a couple of slices of fresh ginger. If you cannot find ginseng, you can use 30g of Radix Codonopsitis Pilosulae (*Dang Shen*) cooked with 50g of white rice in water. Remove the codonopsis at the end and eat the resulting porridge.

For heart blood-spleen qi vacuity depression, cook 100g of white rice with 50g of Semen Coicis Lachryma-jobi (*Yi Yi Ren*) and 10 red dates (Fructus Zizyphi Jujubae, *Da Zao*). Or cook 100g of white rice in chicken broth plus 10 red dates and eat this for dinner every evening for a number of days.

For depression accompanied by insomnia and anxiety due to blood and yin vacuity, use 15g of either Semen Biota Orientalis (*Bai Zi Ren*) or Semen Ziziphi Spinosae (*Suan Zao Ren*) with 100g of white rice and again cook with enough water to make a thin porridge or gruel. Or simply eat cream of wheat every evening before bed instead of dessert.

For depression accompanied by phlegm confounding or blocking the portals of the heart, try cooking 5g of powdered Rhizoma Acori Graminei (*Shi Chang Pu*) with 50g of white rice in water.

For numerous other Chinese medicinal porridge formulas for depression, see my (BF) book, *The Book of Jook: Chinese Medicinal Porridges: A Healthy Alternative to the Typical Western Breakfast* also published by Blue Poppy Press.

Chinese medicinal teas

Chinese medicinal teas may be seen as either Chinese herbal medicine or as Chinese dietary therapy. They consist of using only one or two Chinese herbal medicinals in order to make a tea which is then drunk as one's beverage throughout the day. Such Chinese medicinal teas are usually easier to make and better tasting than multi-ingredient, professionally prescribed decoctions. They can be used as an adjunct to professional prescribed Chinese herbs or as an adjunct to acupuncture or other Chinese therapies for depression.

For liver depression qi stagnation, take 100-150g of fresh plums and add to 320ml of water in a pot and boil for three minutes. Then add 2g of green tea and 25g of honey and steep for 10 minutes. Take one dose in the morning and another dose in the evening. This formula is especially effective for abdominal distention and epigastric oppression associated with liver depression. Another easy tea for liver depression qi stagnation can be made by boiling 25g each of Fructus Immaturus Citri Aurantii (*Zhi Shi*) and Pericarpium Citri Reticulatae (*Chen Pi*) in water for several minutes. Then add 2g of green tea and steep for 10 minutes. Drink the resulting tea as a beverage any time during the day. Yet another tea for liver depression qi stagnation may be made by taking 10g of Tuber Curcumae (*Yu Jin*), *i.e.*, turmeric, and boiling it in one liter of water with 5g of Radix Glycyrrhizae (*Gan Cao*), *i.e.*, licorice. Then add 2g of green tea and a little honey to taste. Drink this as a beverage throughout the day.

For liver depression/depressive heat, boil 30g each of green tea and Fructus Gardeniae Jasminoidis (*Shan Zhi Zi*) in one quart of water and boil until the liquid is reduced by half. Remove the dregs and drink one cup of this liquid in the morning and another in the evening. Or one can take 15g of Flos Chrysanthemi Morifolii (*Ju Hua*) and steep this with 2g of green tea in boiling water for 10 minutes. Then drink the resulting tea as a beverage throughout the day. In addition, jasmine tea purchased at Asian specialty food shops is a good background beverage for those with liver depression with or without heat.

For spleen vacuity fatigue and lack of strength, boil 8g of Radix Panacis Ginseng (*Ren Shen*) for an hour or more in eight ounces of water. Drink this as a tea throughout the day. Asian specialty food stores often sell small porcelain ginseng cookers. These are lidded cups meant to be placed in a pan of water to create a small double-cooker. Basically, the longer you cook ginseng, the more you get out of it. As a substitute for ginseng, you can use double the amount of Radix Codonopsitis Pilosulae (*Dang Shen*). *Do not use ginseng if you suffer from hypertension or high blood pressure.* However, it is much more common to find depression and chronic fatigue occurring in those with hypotension or low blood pressure.

If you suffer from spleen qi and heart blood vacuity, you can try making a tea from 9g of Radix Pseudostellariae (*Tai Zi Shen*), and 15g of Semen Levis Tritici Aestivi (*Fu Xiao Mai*). Place both of these ingredients in a thermos and steep in boiling water for 20 minutes. Then drink as a tea throughout the day. Or you can use 5-10 pieces of Arillus Euphoriae Longanae (*Long Yan Rou*). Place these dried fruits in a double boiler or pressure cooker and steam thoroughly. Then put them in a teacup and steep in boiling water for 10 minutes. Drink the resulting liquid as a tea. Yet another possibility is to boil 10 pieces of Fructus Zizyphi Jujubae (*Da Zao*) in water until the fruit are thoroughly cooked (*i.e.*, completely soft). Then use the resulting liquid to steep 5g of green tea. Drink this as a tea any time throughout the day.

For depression due to heart yin and blood vacuity, grind 15g of Semen Biotae Orientalis (*Bai Zi Ren*) into pieces. Boil with water for 10 minutes and add honey to taste. Drink either before or after dinner. Or boil 15g of Fructus Mori Albi (*Sang Zhen*) in water. Remove the dregs and drink one packet per day. Another option is to grind into powder equal amounts of Fructus Schisandrae Chinensis (*Wu Wei Zi*) and Fructus Lycii Chinensis (*Gou Qi Zi*). Then use 5g of this powder steeped in boiling water for 10 minutes as a tea throughout the day. Or you may use 9g of Semen Zizyphi Spinosae (*Suan Zao Ren*). Pound these into pieces, steep in boiling water for 10 minutes, and drink throughout the day.

For phlegm obstruction with liver depression/depressive heat, grind Rhizoma Acori Graminei (*Shi Chang Pu*), 6g, Flos Jasmini (*Mo Li Hua*), 6g, and green tea, 10g, into coarse powder. Soak some of this powder in boiling water and drink as a tea any time of the day. (You can also use jasmine tea bought at an Asian specialty food shop.) Another formula for phlegm obstruction disturbing the heart spirit but without the heat consists of Dens Draconis (*Long Chi*), 10g, and Rhizoma Acori Graminei (*Shi Chang Pu*), 3g. First boil the Dens Draconis in water for 10 minutes. Then add the Rhizoma Acori Graminei and continue boiling for another 10-15 minutes. Remove the dregs and drink any time of the day, 1-2 packets per day. The doses given are for a one day's supply.

For fire disturbing the heart spirit characterized by restlessness and insomnia, vexation and agitation, a red tongue tip, sores on the tip of the tongue, and heart palpitations, one can boil 60g each of Medulla Junci Effusi (*Deng Xin Cao*) and Folium Lophatheri Gracilis (*Dan Zhu Ye*). Remove the dregs and drink the resulting tea warm at any time of the day, one packet per day.

For more information on Chinese medicinal teas, see Zong Xiao-fan and Gary Liscum's *Chinese Medicinal Teas: Simple, Proven, Folk Formulas for Common Diseases & Promoting Health* also published by Blue Poppy Press.

The medicinals in all the formulas in this chapter can be purchased by mail from:

China Herb Co.
165 W. Queen Lane
Philadelphia, PA 19144
Tel: 215-843-5864
Fax: 215-849-3338
Orders: 800-221-4372

Mayway Corp.
1338 Mandela Parkway
Oakland, CA 94607
Tel: 510-208-3113
Orders: 800-2-Mayway
Fax: 510-208-3069
Orders by fax: 800-909-2828

Flower therapy

People have been giving other people flowers for millennia to help them feel good. In Chinese medicine, there is actually a practice of flower therapy. Because the beauty of flowers bring most people joy and because joy is the antidote to the other four or six negative emotions of Chinese medicine,[18] flowers can help promote the free and easy flow of qi. It is said in Chinese medicine that, "Joy leads to relaxation (in the flow of qi)", and relaxation is exactly what the doctored ordered in case of insomnia. As Wu Shi-ji wrote in the Qing dynasty, "Enjoying flowers can divert a person from their boredom and alleviate suffering caused by the seven affects (or emotions)."

However, there is more to Chinese flower therapy than the beauty of flowers bringing joy. Flower therapy also includes aromatherapy. A number of Chinese medicinals come from plants which have flowers used in bouquets. For instance, Chrysanthemum flowers (*Ju Hua*, Flos Chrysanthemi Morifolii) are used to calm the liver and clear depressive heat rising to the upper body. The aroma of Chrysanthemum flowers thus also has a salutary, relaxing, and cooling effect on liver depression and depressive heat. Rose (*Mei Gui Hua*, Flos Rosae Rugosae) is used in Chinese medicine to move the qi and quicken the blood. Smelling the fragrance of Roses also does these same things. Other flowers used in Chinese medicine to calm the spirit and relieve stress and irritability are Lily, Narcissus, Lotus flowers, Orchids, and Jasmine. And further, taking a smell of a bouquet of flowers promotes deep breathing, and this, in turn, relieves pent up qi in the chest at the same time as it promotes the flow of qi downward via the lungs.

---

[18] In Chinese medicine, the emotions are sometimes counted as five and sometimes counted as seven. When counted as seven, fright and melancholy are added to anger, joy, thinking, sorrow, and fear.

Light therapy

Light therapy, more specifically sunbathing or heliotherapy, is one of Chinese medicine's health preservation and longevity practices. Sunlight is considered the most essential yang qi in nature. Li Shizhen, one of the most famous Chinese doctors of the late Ming dynasty (1368-1644 CE) wrote, "*Tai yang* (literally, supreme yang but a name for the sun) is true fire." As he pointed out, "Without fire, heaven is not able to engender things, and without fire, people are not able to live." Because the back of the human body is yang (as compared to the front which is more yin), exposing the back to sunlight is a good way of increasing one's yang qi.

As we have seen above, most women's yang qi begins to decline by around 35 years of age. In women over 35 years of age, most premenstrual fatigue, loose stools, lack of strength, poor memory, lack of concentration, poor coordination, decline in or lack of libido, low back and knee soreness and weakness, increased nighttime urination, and cold hands and feet are due to this decline first in the yang qi of the spleen and later in the yang qi of the spleen and kidneys. In addition, the spleen qi and kidney yang decline inevitably in both men and women as they get older. Therefore, a decline in the spleen and kidneys is a part of many older people's depression. In such cases, sunbathing can help supplement the yang qi of the body, thereby strengthening the spleen and/or kidneys.

However, because the yang qi is also the motivating force which pushes the qi, increasing yang qi can also help resolve depression and move stagnation. Cao Ting-dong, a famous doctor of the Qing dynasty (1644-1911 CE) wrote:

> Sitting with the back exposed directly to the sun, the back may get warmed. This is able to make the entire body harmonious and smoothly flowing. The sun is the essence of *tai yang* and its light strengthens the yang qi of the human body.

134

In Chinese medicine, whenever the words harmonious and smoothly flowing are used together, they refer to the flow of qi and blood. Hence sun bathing can help course the liver and rectify the qi as well as fortify the spleen and invigorate the kidneys.

It has been said that sunlight is good for every disease except skin cancer. As we now know, overexposure to the sun can cause skin cancer due to sunlight damaging the cells of the skin. Therefore, one should be careful not to get too much sun and not to get burnt. In Chinese medicine, sun bathing should be done between the hours of 8-10 AM. One should only sun bathe between 11 AM-1 PM in winter in temperate, not tropical, latitudes. In addition, we believe that wearing a sun screen of SPF 15 or higher will not lessen the therapeutic warming effects of sun bathing from a Chinese medical point of view.

It is interesting to note that some Western researchers are coming to understand that exposure to light does play a role in many women's PMS as well as in seasonal affection depressive disorder (SADD).

Creating a personalized regime

One does not need to do all these home treatments for every case of depression. Rather, one should select several of them as the severity of their disease, time, and personal inclination suggest. If one is already taking care of the Three Free Therapies, it is easy to add Chinese aromatherapy, Chinese magnet therapy, Chinese flower therapy, and a choice of Chinese medicinal teas, wines, and/or porridges. If one does not have access to body magnets, then one might choose Chinese self-massage therapy. If one doesn't have the patience or discipline to do Chinese self-massage, but a partner is willing to do seven star hammering, then one might choose this therapy instead of self-massage. In other words, it all depends on how severe the depression is and what materials one has at one's disposal.

135

Given the several different Chinese self-therapies in this chapter, no one should be unable to find the materials or the time to put at least one of these into practice. In some light cases of depression, that may be all it takes. While in more difficult, stubborn cases, one may have to do a couple or three of these to insure a good night's sleep without side effects or morning after grogginess.

Additional Suggestions from Clinical Experience

Letting negative thoughts & feelings be

Often, people who are experiencing a depressive episode are unclear about the issues which precipitated the depression in the first place. All has become part of a confused mass of unhappiness, unsettlement, and discomfort. Other times, especially in cases where people have spent considerable time analyzing or processing their situation, the causes and triggering factors are clearly known and understood, yet one doesn't seem to be able to cut through the experience of being depressed.

In such cases, a great deal of energy is spent fighting the anger, frustration, disappointment, and exhaustion that frequently underlie depression. We react to uncomfortable feelings in a similar way in which we react to pain. We constrict, close down, and squeeze in, trying to protect ourselves from the hurt. This is why we have recommended deep relaxation therapy above and why such deep relaxation needs to be somatic, bodily relaxation, and not just mental relaxation. However, when it comes to mental relaxation, it is important to develop an ability to simply let things be as they are. Fighting with our thoughts and emotions does not help. But if we allow them the space to be as they are, they will, by themselves, transform into something else.

According to Asian philosophy, whether it is Buddhism, Confucianism, or Taoism, our thoughts and emotions are like clouds in the sky. Sometimes the sky is full of clouds. Those clouds may be white or grey or black. They may be low or high. They may be thick or thin. They may even be filled with thunder, lightning, and torrential rain. Other times, the sky is cloudless and filled with sunlight. Clouds come and go. But no matter how many or what kind of clouds there are, they never harm, touch, sully, or diminish the essential nature of the space within which they move.

Based on this analogy, it makes little sense to battle with our thoughts and emotions. They come unbidden and they depart without our leave. Good thoughts and pleasurable emotions are supplanted by bad thoughts and painful feelings, but none of these remain forever, *and none of them ever touch or stain our essential nature.* Therefore, when we are overwhelmed with negative emotions, guilt, self-loathing, fear, and doubt, it is best if we simply acknowledge these and let them be. The more we comment on them and try to push them about, the more we simply perpetuate them. Instead, if we simply note their arising, relax our muscular tension, and keep breathing, we will find that, like dew on the morning grass, they have immediately disappeared. In other words, it is best to let your thoughts and emotions be, like clouds in the sky, realizing that ultimately they do not, cannot touch us.

Finding purpose and meaning in one's life

That being said, it is also widely believed in Asia that true happiness comes from doing what needs to be done despite how you may feel about it at the moment. Honora Lee Wolfe, in her book *Second Spring: A Guide to Healthy Menopause with Traditional Chinese Medicine* also published by Blue Poppy Press, recommends women to find some purpose and meaning in life which is greater than one's own. I (RS) find this to be extremely helpful to people experiencing depression, both men and women. Of course, getting up and doing something, even something useful and important, seems impossible in the midst of a depressive episode when you are feeling hopeless and helpless and have lost all sense of meaning and direction. However, once you have overcome the initial phase of a depressive episode, you will hopefully find the strength and inspiration to continue. Finding such purpose and meaning through social, political, ecological, artistic, or spiritual activities helps one overcome momentary setbacks and temporary negative feelings. When one is focused on a goal which is larger than oneself, it is easier to rise to the occasion and, like an elephant walking through the jungle, plod forward step by step no matter what is in front of you. Meaningful activity is the root of self-esteem, and doing what needs to be done next is a sure route to success.

A word about combining psychotherapy with Chinese medicine

In cases where a long history of psychological trauma underlies a person's tendency towards depression, we do recommend that acupuncture and Chinese medicine be combined with psychotherapy by a qualified therapist. As a rule, professional practitioners of Chinese medicine are not qualified to conduct psychotherapy. Yet such psychotherapy can help speed the healing process as well as identify and effectively deal with any crises, such as thoughts of suicide. Therefore, it is in the interest of both the patient and their Chinese medical practitioner to work in combination with a professional psychotherapist.

Conversely, acupuncture not only assists the process of psychotherapy, but, in my experience (RS), it greatly enhances the depth and scope of therapy and helps expedite progress. Many people who have repeatedly worked on their issues in therapy make a forward leap in that therapy when they start acupuncture treatment.

139

Kicking the Antidepressant Habit

Some readers may be currently using Western antidepressants. It is not a good idea to discontinue such medications abruptly without checking with your Western physician. Your Western physician will be able to tell you whether or not you can stop taking a medication immediately or whether it needs to be tapered off at a certain schedule.

It is best if your Western M.D. and your Chinese medical practitioner can work hand in hand. Therefore, if you are currently taking any Western medication, it is important to tell your Chinese medical practitioner what you are taking. In general, there is no problem with taking Western antidepressants with Chinese medicinals or at the same time as receiving acupuncture for depression. If anything, the Chinese medical treatment will make the Western medicines work better and with less side effects. What you should notice fairly quickly is that you need to take less and less of your Western medications to overcome your depressive feelings and your particular symptoms associated with depression. Thus acupuncture and Chinese medicinals can actually help you get off Western antidepressants at the same time as addressing the root of your depression.

In particular, ear acupuncture has been used all over the U.S. to help people kick drug and alcohol addictions. Because press needles can be embedded in the ear between regularly scheduled office visits, this technique allows the calming therapy of acupuncture to exert a continuous effect. Therefore, using ear acupuncture, one can typically avoid any rebound jitters or nervousness when cutting down or stopping taking Western antidepressants.

However, readers who may be suffering from severe mental problems, such as schizophrenia or bipolar disorder (a.k.a. manic depressive disorder), *should not stop taking their Western medication.* Acupuncture and Chinese medicine may help relieve any unwanted side effects from such Western medication, but they typically are not sufficient by themselves for treating such sever mental-emotional problems. Likewise, anyone suffering from severe depression with any thoughts of suicide should immediately seek help from a qualified Western physician or psychotherapist. When using any Chinese medicinal in any form, if there are any side effects, stop immediately and seek a consultation with a professional practitioner of Chinese medicine.

A Controlled Study of Acupuncture in the Treatment of Depression

In 1993, the Office of Alternative Medicine (OAM) of the National Institutes of Health (NIH) funded 30 exploratory grants to encourage collaboration between conventional researchers and practitioners of alternative medicine. The purpose of these grants was to conduct small-scale preliminary studies to investigate whether some alternative therapies may warrant further study in the treatment of certain conditions.

In collaboration with John J. B. Allen, Ph.D., a professor of Clinical Psychology at the University of Arizona in Tucson, I (RS) designed a study of acupuncture in the treatment of depression in women. The aim of our study was not only to determine the efficacy of acupuncture in treating depression but also to explore Chinese medicine's individualized treatment approach within the framework of established scientific research protocols. We were fortunate to be one of the 30 studies initially funded by the OAM and one of only two to study acupuncture.

Because the dollar amounts of these grants were very small compared to typical grants made by the NIH for "conventional" medical research, we were forced to narrow our focus to a particular group of patients within the larger population of all possible sufferers of depression. However, based on my clinical experience and supported by statistical data, it is members of this group who suffer most commonly from depression. I am talking about women 18-45 years of age.

Description of the Study

Thirty-eight women aged 18-45 were recruited through newspaper ads. These ads offered "non-drug" treatment for depression but did not mention acupuncture. The participants were first interviewed over the phone to see if they met our exclusion criteria. In other words, women suffering from dysthymia, chronic depression, bipolar disorder, a history of psychosis or mania, or other current clinical psychiatric disorders were excluded. Any women with substance abuse or dependency within the past four months, who were undergoing current treatment for depression (psychotherapy or pharmacotherapy), or who had endocrine abnormalities (thyroid disorder, Addison's diseases, etc.), lesions of the central nervous system, or seizure disorders, or who were pregnant were also excluded. In addition, women who presented with an active potential for suicide were excluded as well.

Study Design

After the phone interview, those women who met the criteria for the study received a SCID interview (Structural Clinical Interview). This is a standard psychological interview to determine if they meet the DSM-IV (*Diagnostic Manual of Mental Disorders*, 4th edition) criteria for major depression. This interview was conducted by masters level qualified psychologists.

A traditional Chinese medical diagnosis was then conducted by an acupuncturist to determine their Chinese pattern discrimination, treatment principles, and acupuncture treatment plan. These treatments were designed by the assessing acupuncturist but were administered by four other acupuncturists. Neither the assessing acupuncturist nor the treating acupuncturists knew which treatment group the patient was in.

Participants were assigned to one of three groups: specific, non-specific, and wait-list. Patients assigned to the specific group each received acupuncture treatment specifically to treat depression. Patients assigned to the nonspecific group received treatment for their Chinese pattern of disharmony but which did not address depression directly. Patients assigned to the wait-list group waited before receiving specific treatment. All treatments were tailored to the individual and were based on Chinese medical patterrn discrimination.

The specific group received eight weeks of specific treatment. The nonspecific group received eight weeks of nonspecific treatment and then eight weeks of specific treatment. While the wait-list group waited eight weeks and then received eight weeks of specific treatment. Each eight week segment consisted of 12 sessions: two sessions per week for four weeks; then one session per week for four more weeks. By the end of this study, all participants had received specific treatment to address their pattern of disharmony as it related to their depression.

In addition to the SCID interview at the beginning of the study, participants were also administered the Hamilton Rating Scale for Depression (HRSD) before treatment began and again after four and eight weeks in the specific treatment group and, in addition, after 12 and 16 weeks in the nonspecific and wait-list treatment groups. Patients also filled out self-report forms. Alliance to the therapist and resistance to treatment were also measured.

Study Results

After completion of the specific treatment, using the DSM-IV remission criteria, 64% of the women experienced full remission, 18% of the women experienced partial remission, and 18% experienced no remission. Using the Hamilton Rating Scale as the criterion for remission, 70% of all women experienced remission, while 30% did not. These results compare favorably to both psychotherapy and pharmacotherapy whose effectiveness falls between 65-70%. The drop-out rate was only 13% in the acupuncture study compared to over 30% of most other studies.

145

Specific acupuncture treatment produced a significant reduction of symptoms over time and it demonstrated greater reduction in symptoms over eight weeks than the nonspecific group. However, it did not demonstrate a significantly greater reduction than the wait-list group.

Conclusions

These preliminary findings suggest that *acupuncture is as effective as pharmacotherapy or psychotherapy as a treatment for depression.* In addition, this study is a first attempt at conducting research according to established research protocols while respecting the individualized nature of Chinese medicine. It indicates that people who suffer from depression benefit from acupuncture treatment per se and not just because they expect to get better or because they derive benefit from interacting with a therapist on a weekly basis.

What does this research mean for sufferers of depression?

Due to the limited nature of the study, the sample of women included was very small. Therefore, these findings are clearly preliminary. A larger scale study with many more women corroborating our findings will be necessary before acupuncture will be recognized as a viable treatment for depression by the scientific community. Nevertheless, this study does suggest that acupuncture is just as effective for the treatment of depression as psychotherapy and drug therapy. Since acupuncture as a part of Chinese medicine seeks to rebalance the health of the entire organism, body *and* mind, we feel that the total healing impact of this treatment is greater than that of either psychotherapy or drug therapy alone. In addition, professionally administered acupuncture has no or extremely minimal side effects (occasional black and blue marks). Therefore, we think that people suffering from depression should consider acupuncture and Chinese medicine as either an alternative or complement to conventional Western therapy.

More Case Histories

In order to help readers get a better feel for how Chinese medicine treats depression, we have given below some more case histories. These are the stories of real-life people who I (RS) have treated with acupuncture and/or Chinese medicine for depression and gotten a good effect. Hopefully, you will be able to see yourself and your symptoms in these stories and be encouraged to give acupuncture and Chinese medicine a try.

Adrianna

Adrianna was 27 years old. When she sought treatment with Chinese medicine she was currently on medication for depression and anxiety. She wanted to start a family and didn't want to continue on medication. She had been told by her physician that, given her tendency towards recurrent depression and her family history of depression, she needed to stay on antidepressants for the rest of her life. She was determined to find an alternative.

At the onset of this last episode, Adrianna had been under a lot of stress due to numerous life changes. She felt lethargic, had trouble concentrating, felt withdrawn, and couldn't interact socially. She felt emotionally and physically drained and cried constantly. Her appetite was erratic, she felt bloated, was nauseous, and experienced diarrhea during stressful events. She felt tired all the time, yet she couldn't sleep well and would wake up regularly through the night. Her thoughts raced constantly and she felt anxious and restless.

Adrianna had been on birth control pills for five years and had just gone off them a few months after the onset of her depression. She had a history of long cycles, inconsistent, dark flow, and cramping both at ovulation and during her period. Premenstrually, she experienced abdominal bloating, breast distention, low backache, leg pain, acne on her face, upper back, and chest areas, and a worsening of her depressive symptoms. At the time I first saw Adrianna, she had not had a period for several months.

On examination, Adrianna's tongue was very puffy but dark and had a thin, frothy, white coating, especially on the sides. Her pulse was bowstring and a bit rapid but very deep and weak in the third or proximal positions on both sides.[19]

Adrianna's Chinese medical pattern discrimination as I read it was liver depression qi stagnation and slight depressive heat affecting the heart with underlying spleen qi vacuity, damp accumulation, and possibly kidney vacuity. Therefore the treatment principles were to course the liver and rectify the qi, clear heat and resolve depression while fortifying the spleen and transforming dampness. If, as treatment progressed, kidney yang vacuity became more evident, it would be addressed accordingly. Because her period had not come for several months and because of some of her specific menstrual symptoms, the principles of quickening the blood and regulating the menses were added to her treatment plan. Adrianna was given the following Chinese medical prescription:

Radix Bupleuri *(Chai Hu),* 9g
Radix Scutellariae Baicalensis *(Huang Qin),* 9g
Radix Panacis Ginseng *(Ren Shen),* 9g

---

[19] Chinese medical practitioners read three longitudinal positions on the radial arteries at the wrists. These are called the inch, bar, and cubit. The inch is the most distal (*i.e.*, distant from the torso), the bar is directly over the styloid process, and the cubit is the most proximal (*i.e.*, is closest to the torso). The inch corresponds to the upper body, the bar corresponds to the area of the body between the diaphragm and the navel, and the cubit corresponds to the lower body.

Rhizoma Pinelliae Ternatae *(Ban Xia)*, 4.5g
mix-fried Radix Glycyrrhizae *(Gan Cao)*, 4.5g
uncooked Rhizoma Zingiberis *(Sheng Jiang)*, 3g
Radix Angelicae Sinensis *(Dang Gui)*, 4.5g
Radix Ligustici Wallichii *(Chuang Xiong)*, 9g
Rhizoma Cyperi Rotundi *(Xiang Fu)*, 9g
Sclerotium Poriae Cocos *(Fu Ling)*, 6g
Radix Polygalae Tenuifoliae *(Yuan Zhi)*, 6g
Semen Zizyphi Spinosae *(Suan Zao Ren)*, 6g

The above Chinese medicinals were decocted in water and administered in two divided doses per day after breakfast and lunch. In addition, Adrianna received regular acupuncture sessions once a week. Some of the points used in her acupuncture sessions were:

Tai Chong (Liv 3)   *Gong Sun* (Sp 4)
He Gu (LI 4)   *Nei Guan* (Per 6)
Zhong Wan (CV 12)   *San Yin Jiao* (Sp 6)

She was able to decrease her medication gradually, both the antidepressant and the antianxiety medications, until she was able to discontinue them completely. After taking the decoction for three weeks, she continued with the acupuncture sessions for several more weeks, tapering off to maintenance treatments once a month. Adrianna was instructed to diminish her consumption of wheat and dairy products, eliminate sweets from her diet, and exercise regularly as well as develop a relaxation routine. She no longer feels depressed, sleeps soundly through the night, and is preparing to start a family. Adrianna's cycles have become more regular and she has experienced a decrease of premenstrual symptoms.

Elana

Elana was 47 years old. She had experienced the loss of three very significant people in her life in the past several months. She had

151

been clinically diagnosed with depression two weeks prior to her first visit. Upon questioning, I found out that she had experienced severe depressive episodes a few times in the course of her life. She was now on an antidepressant and was experiencing uncomfortable side effects and still felt depressed. She had nightmares and crying spells, felt hopeless, and was very sad most of the time. Her appetite was erratic, she burped constantly, she was constipated, and she had a history of gastric ulcers. Elana felt irritable and extremely anxious. She couldn't calm herself down and periodically erupted angrily at the people around her. She still had regular periods. However, these were becoming shorter in duration, scantier in amount, and were a bit clotty. She had no significant premenstrual symptoms. Her pulse was slippery, rapid, and bowstring on both sides. Her tongue was swollen and reddish with a thick, yellowish white coating. Elana's Chinese medical pattern differentiation as I saw it was phlegm heat internally harassing with concomitant liver depression. The Chinese medicinal prescription I recommended for her was composed of:

Rhizoma Pinelliae Ternatae *(Ban Xia),* 9g
Sclerotium Poriae Cocos *(Fu Ling),* 9g
mix-fried Radix Glycyrrhizae *(Gan Cao),* 4.5g
Pericarpium Citri Reticulatae *(Chen Pi),* 9g
uncooked Rhizoma Zingiberis *(Sheng Jiang),* 3g
Caulis Bambusae In Taeniis *(Zhu Ru),* 9g
Fructus Immaturus Citri Aurantii *(Zhi Shi),* 9g
Fructus Zizyphi Jujubae *(Da Zao),* 3g
Rhizoma Coptis Chinensis *(Huan Lian),* 3g
Semen Ziziphi Spinosae *(Suan Zao Ren),* 4.5g
Rhizoma Acori Graminei *(Shi Chang Pu),* 4.5g
Radix Salviae Miltiorrhizae *(Dan Shen),* 6g
Tuber Curcumae *(Yu Jin),* 4.5g
Radix Polygalae Tenuifoliae *(Yuan Zhi),* 4.5g

Elana discontinued the antidepressants and took the ingredients of this formula for two weeks in decoction form. Then, due to traveling and her busy schedule, she discontinued the decoction but continued on two formulas in tablet form which combined most of the above mentioned ingredients. She called the office several weeks later to ask for a refill of the tablets and reported she was feeling very well. She no longer felt depressed, she was sleeping well, and she no longer felt irritable and anxious. In addition, all her digestive problems had completely disappeared.

Robert

Robert was 52 years old. He was feeling extremely hopeless and sad. He was very critical of himself and had a very poor self-image. He felt exhausted at the end of the day and had difficulty catching up after a long day of work. He also cried easily. Because this was extremely embarrassing in front of his friends, he had become isolated. All these conditions had become more evident in the last couple of years after a long-term relationship had ended. Robert had been on antidepressants briefly a few months previously, but he didn't want to go back on medication. He felt nauseous a lot, had no appetite, and described a sinking feeling in his chest. This was accompanied by breathlessness, sighing, and a sensation of something stuck in his throat. He experienced frequent night time urination and had lower backache. His tongue was very swollen and pale with a slight purplish tinge and a wet, thin, white coating. Robert's pulse was slightly slippery but mostly weak and empty.

My reading of Robert's Chinese medical pattern differentiation was spleen-kidney yang vacuity giving rise to phlegm dampness obstruction and stagnation. Therefore, the treatment principles were to fortify the spleen and invigorate the kidneys, downbear counterflow and transform phlegm. Based on these principles, I gave Robert a decoction which included the following ingredients:

Rhizoma Pinelliae Ternata (Ban Xia), 12g
Cortex Magnoliae Officinalis (Huo Po), 9g
Folium Perillae Frutescentis (Zi Su Ye), 6g
Sclerotium Poriae Cocos (Fu Ling), 9g
Fructus Zizyphi Jujubae (Da Zao), 4.5g

uncooked Rhizoma Zingiberis *(Sheng Jiang)*, 3g
Radix Panacis Ginseng *(Ren Shen)*, 9g
Rhizoma Atractylodis Macrocephalae *(Bai Zhu)*, 6g
Cortex Cinnamomi Cassiae *(Rou Gui)*, 4.5g
Cortex Eucommiae Ulmoidis *(Du Zhong)*, 6g
Semen Cuscutae Chinensis *(Tu Si Zi)*, 6g
Radix Bupleuri *(Chai Hu)*, 4.5g
Pericarpium Citri Reticulatae Viride *(Qing Pi)*, 4.5g

Robert took the prescription above as a decoction, two times per day. In addition, he was instructed to limit his intake of uncooked foods and cold drinks and to begin a sensitive exercise program. He also received five acupuncture sessions, which consisted on needling the following points:

Pi Shu (Bl 20)	*Dan Zhong* (CV 17)
Shen Shu (Bl 23)	*Nei Guan* (Per 6)
Feng Long (St 40)	*Tai Chong* (Liv 3)
Lie Que (Lu 7)	*Tai Xi* (Ki 3)

After beginning with the above treatments, Robert reported feeling much more energetic and enthusiastic. He began volunteering at his local community center. His appetite improved, he no longer woke up at night to urinate, and his back didn't hurt as often.

Carmen

Carmen was 35 years old. She had experienced low-grade depression for as long as she could remember. Lately, she felt stuck, had no interest in anything, and was having a lot of difficulty making decisions. She felt guilty a lot of the time and alternated between being extremely fatigued and overly irritable. Carmen said that she had always felt like an outsider in her own world. She has a history of chronic constipation, her appetite was not very good, her hair was limp, her skin and lips were very dry, and she experienced heart palpitations. Her menstrual cycles were long and her periods were scanty, a bit dark, and clotty. Premenstrually, she had sharp breast pain, increased irritability, and difficulty falling asleep. Her tongue was puffy and pale but darker on the sides and tip. Her pulse was bowstring and very fine.

Carmen's Chinese medical pattern differentiation was liver depression qi stagnation with blood vacuity. The treatment principles were to course the liver and rectify the qi, nourish the liver and supplement the blood. Carmen was given a decoction which consisted of the following ingredients:

Radix Bupleuri (*Chai Hu*), 7.5g
Radix Angelicae Sinensis (*Dang Gui*), 9g
Radix Albus Paeoniae Lactiflorae (*Bai Shao*), 9g
Rhizoma Atractylodis Macrocephalae (*Bai Zhu*), 6g
Sclerotium Poriae Cocos (*Fu Ling*), 6g
mix-fried Radix Glycyrrhizae (*Gan Cao*), 4.5g
Herba Menthae Haplocalycis (*Bo He*), 3g
uncooked Rhizoma Zingiberis (*Sheng Jiang*), 3g
Fructus Lycii Chinensis *(Gou Ci Zi)*, 6g
Semen Biotae Orientalis *(Bai Zi Ren)*, 4.5g
Cortex Albizziae Julibrissinis *(He Huan Pi)*, 4.5g

In addition, Carmen was instructed to include a bit more animal protein in her diet, while minimizing uncooked and chilled foods. After taking the decoction for four weeks, Carmen's cycle was not long like it had been. Instead, it came precisely at 28 days. She experienced very little premenstrual discomfort, was able to fall asleep easily, and had no breast pain. In addition, Carmen gained enough confidence to change jobs and terminate a relationship that was no longer nurturing to her.

Alan

Alan was 45 years old and was an important executive of a large firm. He had always been able to work hard and for long hours and to meet deadlines. Alan was proud of making personal sacrifices for the success of his company. Lately, however, he had been extremely

155

hostile towards his coworkers. He became annoyed and frustrated easily. Further, Alan said he had lost interest in his job, had no contact with his friends, and had withdrawn from his family. After working 12-15 hours a day, he drank heavily and collapsed on the weekend. He felt a feeling of tightness and oppression in his chest, sighed frequently, and felt tired all the time. He often woke in the middle of the night with nightmares. People close to Alan had made repeated suggestions about his condition, but he was unwilling to consider changing his patterns. After nearly being involved in a head-on collision, Alan decided he needed to do something. His wife suggested he try acupuncture.

When Alan came in for his first visit with me, his tongue was dark and reddish and had a frothy, white coating on the center towards the sides. His pulse was extremely bowstring and rapid. Based on these signs and all the symptoms he reported to me above, Alan's Chinese medical pattern discrimination was liver depression qi stagnation which had progressed into depressed and bound heat, dampness, and blood. The treatment principles, therefore, were to course the liver and rectify the qi, clear heat and resolve depression, transform dampness and quicken the blood. Based on these principles, the Chinese medicinal formula I chose for Alan was composed of the following ingredients:

Rhizoma Cyperi Rotundi *(Xiang Fu)*, 9g
Radix Ligustici Wallichii *(Chiang Xiong)*, 6g
Fructus Gardeniae Jasminoidis *(Zhi Zi)*, 6g
Rhizoma Atractylodis *(Cang Zhu)*, 6g
Massa Medica Fermentata *(Shen Qu)*, 4.5g
Rhizoma Acori Graminei *(Shi Chang Pu)*, 4.5g
Tuber Curcumae *(Yu Jin)*, 4.5g
Rhizoma Coptidis Chinensis *(Huan Lian)*, 3g

In addition, Alan received eight acupuncture sessions which consisted of some of the following points:

Xiang Jian (Liv 2)   *Tai Chong* (Liv 3)

He Gu (LI 4)	*Qi Men* (Liv 14)
Qu Chi (LI 11)	*Jiu Wei* (CV 15)
Da Ling (Per 7)	*Yin Tang* (M-HN-3)

Alan reported that he felt calmer, more even tempered, and more enthusiastic about his job. He decided to do some short-term cognitive therapy to help him develop strategies to better cope with stress and to learn how to balance work with personal interests and family life. He continued bi-monthy acupuncture sessions for about six months, at the same time as he developed exercise and relaxation routines, and continued trying to limit his time at the office. As of this writing, he no longer feels tightness and oppression in his chest, he sleeps well most of the time, and he is only drinking occasionally at social events.

As the above case histories show, Chinese medicine treats the whole person. It is not just symptomatic treatment. In all the above cases, the patients not only overcame their depression, but other of their symptoms also "miraculously" disappeared. Actually, there is nothing miraculous about it. If these accompanying symptoms had not disappeared, the Chinese doctor would have thought that the treatment was not completely successful.

Although Chinese medicine does not work immediately, because it treats the whole person, it is usually worth the wait and perseverance. Western antidepressants also take some time to beg in acting, but they also usually produce unpleasant side effects. In addition, once one understands that Chinese medicine is not a symptomatic "quick fix", this motivates the person to keep on with a good diet, regular exercise, and daily deep relaxation.

Finding a Professional Practitioner of Chinese Medicine

Traditional Chinese medicine is one of the fastest growing holistic health care systems in the West today. At the present time, there are 50 colleges in the United States alone which offer 3-4 year training programs in acupuncture, moxibustion, Chinese herbal medicine, and Chinese medical massage. In addition, many of the graduates of these programs have done postgraduate studies at colleges and hospitals in China, Taiwan, Hong Kong, and Japan. Further, a growing number of trained Oriental medical practitioners have immigrated from China, Japan, and Korea to practice acupuncture and Chinese herbal medicine in the West.

Traditional Chinese medicine, including acupuncture, is a discreet and independent health care profession. It is not simply a technique that can easily be added to the array of techniques of some other health care profession. The study of Chinese medicine, acupuncture, and Chinese herbs is as rigorous as is the study of allopathic, chiropractic, naturopathic, or homeopathic medicine. Previous training in any one of these other systems does not automatically confer competence or knowledge in Chinese medicine. In order to get the full benefits and safety of Chinese medicine, one should seek out professionally trained and credentialed practitioners.

In the United States, recognition that acupuncture and Chinese medicine are their own independent professions has led to the creation of the National Commission for the Certification of Acupuncture & Oriental Medicine (NCCAOM). This commission has created and administers a national board examination in both

159

acupuncture and Chinese herbal medicine in order to insure minimum levels of professional competence and safety. Those who pass the acupuncture exam append the letters Dipl. Ac. (Diplomate of Acupuncture) after their names, while those who pass the Chinese herbal exam use the letters Dipl. C.H. (Diplomate of Chinese Herbs). I recommend that persons wishing to experience the benefits of acupuncture and Chinese medicine should seek treatment in the U.S. only from those who are NCCAOM certified.

In addition, in the United States, acupuncture is a legal, independent health care profession in more than half the states. A few other states require acupuncturists to work under the supervision of M.D.s, while in a number of states, acupuncture has yet to receive legal status. In states where acupuncture is licensed and regulated, the names of acupuncture practitioners can be found in the *Yellow Pages* of your local phone book or through contacting your State Department of Health, Board of Medical Examiners, or Department of Regulatory Agencies. In states without licensure, it is doubly important to seek treatment only from NCCAOM diplomates.

When seeking a qualified and knowledgeable practitioner, word of mouth referrals are important. Satisfied patients are the most reliable credential a practitioner can have. It is appropriate to ask the practitioner for references from previous patients treated for the same problem. It is best to work with a practitioner who communicates effectively enough for the patient to feel understood and for the Chinese medical diagnosis and treatment plan to make sense. In all cases, a professional practitioner of Chinese medicine should be able and willing to give a written traditional Chinese diagnosis of the patient's pattern upon request.

For further information regarding the practice of Chinese medicine and acupuncture in the United States of America and for referrals to local professional associations and practitioners in the United States, prospective patients may contact:

160

National Commission for the Certification of Acupuncture &
Oriental Medicine
11 Canal Center Plaza, Suite 300
Alexandria, VA 22314
Tel: (703) 548-9004
Fax: (703) 548-9079

The National Acupuncture & Oriental Medicine Alliance
14637 Starr Rd, SE
Olalla, WA 98357
Tel: (206) 851-6895
Fax: (206) 728-4841
email: 76143.2061@compuserve.com

The American Association of Oriental Medicine
433 Front St.
Catasauqua, PA 18032-2506
Tel: (610) 433-2448
Fax: (610) 433-1832

Learning More About Chinese Medicine

For more information on Chinese medicine in general, see:

The Web That Has No Weaver: Understanding Chinese Medicine by Ted Kaptchuk, Congdon & Weed, NY, 1983. This is the best overall introduction to Chinese medicine for the serious lay reader. It has been a standard since it was first published over a dozen years ago and it has yet to be replaced.

Chinese Secrets of Health & Longevity by Bob Flaws, Sound True, Boulder, CO, 1996. This is a six tape audiocassette course introducing Chinese medicine to laypeople. It covers basic Chinese medical theory, Chinese dietary therapy, Chinese herbal medicine, acupuncture, *qi gong, feng shui,* deep relaxation, life-style, and more.

Fundamentals of Chinese Medicine by the East Asian Medical Studies Society, Paradigm Publications, Brookline, MA, 1985. This is a more technical introduction and overview of Chinese medicine intended for professional entry level students.

Traditional Medicine in Contemporary China by Nathan Sivin, Center for Chinese Studies, University of Michigan, Ann Arbor, 1987. This book discusses the development of Chinese medicine in China in the last half century.

Imperial Secrets of Health and Longevity by Bob Flaws, Blue Poppy Press, Inc. Boulder, CO, 1994. This book includes a section on

Chinese dietary therapy and generally introduces the basic concepts of good health according to Chinese medicine.

The Mystery of Longevity by Liu Zheng-cai, Foreign Languages Press, Beijing, 1990. This book is also about general principles and practices promoting good health according to Chinese medicine.

For more information on Chinese dietary therapy, see:

The Tao of Healthy Eating: A Simple Guide to Diet According to Traditional Chinese Medicine by Bob Flaws, Blue Poppy Press, Inc., Boulder, CO, 1997. This book is a layperson's primer on Chinese dietary therapy. It includes detailed sections on the clear, bland diet as well as sections on chronic candidiasis and allergies.

Prince Wen Hui's Cook: Chinese Dietary Therapy by Bob Flaws & Honora Lee Wolfe, Paradigm Publications, Brookline, MA, 1983. This book is an introduction to Chinese dietary therapy. Although some of the information it contains is dated, it does give the Chinese medicinal descriptions of most foods commonly eaten in the West.

The Book of Jook: Chinese Medicinal Porridges, A Healthy Alternative to the Typical Western Breakfast by Bob Flaws, Blue Poppy Press, Inc., Boulder, CO, 1995. This book is specifically about Chinese medicinal porridges made with very simple combinations of Chinese medicinal herbs.

Chinese Medicinal Wines & Elixirs by Bob Flaws, Blue Poppy Press, Inc., Boulder, CO, 1995. This book is a large collection of simple one, two, and three Chinese medicinal wines which can be made at home.

Chinese Medicinal Teas: Simple, Proven Folk Formulas for Treating Disease & Promoting Health by Zong Xiao-fan & Gary Liscum, Blue Poppy Press, Inc., Boulder, CO, 1997. Like the above two books, this

164

book is about one, two, and three ingredient Chinese medicinal teas which are easy to make and can be used at home as adjuncts to other, professionally prescribed treatments or for the promotion of health and prevention of disease.

The Tao of Nutrition by Maoshing Ni, Union of Tao and Man, Los Angeles, 1989. This book is also a good overview of Chinese dietary therapy written specifically for a Western lay audience.

Harmony Rules: The Chinese Way of Health Through Food by Gary Butt & Frena Bloomfield, Samuel Weiser, Inc., York Beach, ME, 1985. This book tries to make Chinese dietary therapy more easily understandable for Western lay readers. Therefore, its discussion of Chinese dietary therapy is not exactly a standard approach. However, it does include much useful information.

Chinese System of Food Cures: Prevention & Remedies by Henry C. Lu, Sterling Publishing Co., Inc, NY, 1986. This book is somewhat more standard. It includes most of the same information found in *The Tao of Nutrition*. We suggest that you pick one or the other of these.

A Practical English-Chinese Library of Traditional Chinese Medicine: Chinese Medicated Diet ed. by Zhang En-qin, Shanghai College of Traditional Chinese Medicine Publishing House, Shanghai, 1990. This is a very standard discussion of Chinese dietary therapy written for professional practitioners. However, it is still understandable by nonprofessional readers.

Eating Your Way to Health—Dietotherapy in Traditional Chinese Medicine by Cai Jing-feng, Foreign Languages Press, Beijing, 1988. This is a slim little book which gives the pith of Chinese dietary therapy. The English is not very good, but the information is certainly OK.

For more information on Chinese patent medicines, see:

Clinical Handbook of Chinese Prepared Medicine by Chun-han Zhu, Paradigm Publications, Brookline, MA, 1989. This book is an excellent reference text for Chinese prepared or so-called patent medicines. It uses a professionally accurate, standard translational terminology similar to that used in this book. So readers of this book should feel comfortable with the terminology in that book. It is beautifully designed and laid out and is easy to use. This is most definitely my first choice of books on Chinese patent medicines.

Outline Guide to Chinese Herbal Patent Medicines in Pill Form by Margaret A. Naeser, Boston Chinese Medicine, Boston, 1990. This book contains basically the same information as the preceding title. However, it is a paperback and is more "home-made" through desk-top publishing. Therefore, it is a cheaper source of essentially the same information in not so nice a package. It also does not use a professionally accurate, standard translational terminology.

For more information on Chinese herbs and formulas, see:

Chinese Herbal Medicine: Materia Medica by Dan Bensky & Andrew Gamble, Eastland Press, Seattle, 1993. This is the "industry standard" when it comes to descriptions of the basic Chinese materia medica. Under each entry you will find the temperature, flavors, channel-enterings, functions, indications, combinations, dosages, and contraindications of all the most important Chinese medicinals.

Chinese Herbal Medicine: Formulas & Strategies by Dan Bensky & Randall Barolet, Eastland Press, Seattle, 1990. This is the companion volume to the preceding text. It is the industry standard for descriptions of all the main Chinese medicinal formulas. Under each entry, it gives the ingredients and their dosages, functions,

166

indications, dosages and administration of the formula as a whole, and cautions and contraindications of all the most important Chinese formulas.

Oriental Materia Medica: A Concise Guide by Hong-yen Hsu *et al.*, Oriental Healing Arts Institute, Long Beach, CA, 1986. This book is a pharmacopeia similar to Bensky & Gamble's above. The information it contains under each herb is not as complete, but it contains many more medicinals. Therefore, it is the next place to look when Bensky & Gamble do not list a particular Chinese medicinal you are trying to find out about.

A Clinical Guide to Chinese Herbs and Formulae by Chen Song Yu & Li Fei, Churchill Livingstone, Edinburgh, 1993. This book contains basic information on both Chinese herbs as individuals, the main Chinese herbal formulas, and the Chinese herbal treatment of the most common diseases with Chinese herbal medicine. Compared to the above books, this book is essentially meant as a textbook for a *course* on Chinese herbal medicine. In that case, the above books become reference texts for the *practice* of Chinese herbal medicine.

Chinese Herbal Remedies by Albert Y. Leung, Universe Books, NY, 1984. This book is about simple Chinese herbal home remedies.

Legendary Chinese Healing Herbs by Henry C. Lu, Sterling Publishing, Inc., NY, 1991. This book is a fun way to begin learning about Chinese herbal medicine. It is full of interesting and entertaining anecdotes about Chinese medicinal herbs.

For more information on Asian insights into psychology & psychotherapy, see:

The Quiet Therapies: Japanese Pathways to Personal Growth, David K. Reynolds, University of Hawaii Press, Honolulu, 1987. This book is a great little introduction to Japanese forms of psychotherapy based on doing, not analyzing. It also talks about the psychotherapeutic benefits of deep relaxation. David Reynolds has since gone on to author a number of other popular books on Asian insights to psychological health, such as *Playing Ball on Running Water* and *Even in Winter the Ice Doesn't Melt*.

Tibetan Buddhist Medicine and Psychiatry: The Diamond Healing, Samuel Weiser Inc., York Beach, ME, 1984. This book explains the Tibetan Buddhist approach to the diagnosis and treatment of mental/emotional disorders. Although Tibetan medicine is not exactly the same as Chinese medicine, they are "kissing cousins" and many of the insights of Tibetan medicine in terms of psychological disorders is very profound and effective.

Chinese Medical Glossary

Chinese medicine is a system unto itself. Its technical terms are uniquely its own and cannot be reduced to the definitions of Western medicine without destroying the very fabric and logic of Chinese medicine. Ultimately, because Chinese medicine was created in the Chinese language, Chinese medicine is best and really only understood in that language. Nevertheless, as Westerners trying to understand Chinese medicine, we must translate the technical terms of Chinese medicine in English words. If some of these technical translations sound at first peculiar and their meaning is not immediately transparent, this is because no equivalent concepts exist in everyday English.

In the past, some Western authors have erroneously translated technical Chinese medical terms using Western medical or at least quasi-scientific words in an attempt to make this system more acceptable to Western audiences. For instance, the words tonify and sedate are commonly seen in the Western Chinese medical literature even though, in the case of sedate, its meaning is 180° opposite to the Chinese understanding of the word *xie*. *Xie* means to drain off something which has pooled and accumulated. That accumulation is seen as something excess which should not be lingering where it is. Because it is accumulating somewhere where it shouldn't, it is impeding and obstructing whatever should be moving to and through that area. The word sedate comes from the Latin word *sedere*, to sit. Therefore, the word sedate means to make something sit still. In English, we get the word sediment from this same root. However, the Chinese *xie* means draining off something which is sitting somewhere erroneously. Therefore, to think that one is going to sedate what is already sitting is a great mistake in understanding the clinical implication and application of this technical term.

Thus, in order, to preserve the integrity of this system while still making it intelligible to English language readers, we have appended the following glossary of Chinese medical technical terms. The terms themselves are based on Nigel Wiseman's *English-Chinese Chinese-English Dictionary of Chinese Medicine* published by the Hunan Science & Technology Press in Changsha, Hunan, People's Republic of China in 1995. Dr. Wiseman is, we believe, the greatest Western scholar in terms of the translation of Chinese medicine into English. As a Chinese reader myself (BF), although I often find Wiseman's terms awkward sounding at first, I also think they convey most accurately the Chinese understanding and logic of these terms.

Acquired essence: Essence manufactured out of the surplus of qi and blood in turn created out of the refined essence of food and drink
Acupoints: Those places on the channels and network vessels where qi and blood tend to collect in denser concentrations, and thus those places where the qi and blood in the channels are especially available for manipulation
Acupuncture: The regulation of qi flow by the stimulation of certain points located on the channels and network vessels achieved mainly by the insertion of fine needles into these points
Aromatherapy: Using various scents and smells to treat and prevent disease
Ascendant hyperactivity of liver yang: Upwardly out of control counterflow of liver yang due to insufficient yin to hold it down in the lower part of the body
Blood: The red colored fluid which flows in the vessels and nourishes and constructs the tissues of the body
Blood stasis: Also called dead blood, malign blood, and dry blood, blood stasis is blood which is no longer moving through the vessels as it should. Instead it is precipitated in the vessels like silt in a river. Like silt, it then obstructs the free flow of the blood in the vessels and also impedes the production of new or fresh blood.

Blood vacuity: Insufficient blood manifesting in diminished nourishment, construction, and moistening of body tissues

Bowels: The hollow yang organs of Chinese medicine

Channels: The main routes for the distribution of qi and blood, but mainly qi

Clear: The pure or clear part of food and drink ingested which is then turned into qi and blood

Counterflow: An erroneous flow of qi, usually upward but sometimes horizontally as well

Dampness: A pathological accumulation of body fluids

Decoction: A method of administering Chinese medicinals by boiling these medicinals in water, removing the dregs, and drinking the resulting medicinal liquid

Depression: Stagnation and lack of movement, as in liver depression qi stagnation

Depressive heat: Pathological heat transformed due to qi depression or stagnation

Drain: To drain off or away some pathological qi or substance from where it is replete or excess

Essence: A stored, very potent form of substance and qi, usually yin when compared to yang qi, but can be transformed into yang qi

Five phase theory: An ancient Chinese system of correspondences dividing up all of reality into five phases of development which then mutually engender and check each other according to definite sequences.

Hydrotherapy: Using various baths and water applications to treat and prevent disease

Life gate fire: Another name for kidney yang or kidney fire, seen as the ultimate source of yang qi in the body.

Magnet therapy: Applying magnets to acupuncture points to treat and prevent disease

Moxibustion: Burning the herb Artemisia Argyium on, over, or near acupuncture points in order to add yang qi, warm cold, or promote the movement of the qi and blood

Network vessels: Small vessels which form a net-like web insuring the flow of qi and blood to all body tissues

Phlegm: A pathological accumulation of phlegm or mucus congealed from dampness or body fluids

Qi: Activity, function, that which moves, transforms, defends, restrains, and warms

Portals: Also called orifices, the openings of the sensory organs and the opening of the heart through which the spirit makes contact with the world outside

Qi mechanism: The process of transforming yin substance controlled and promoted by the qi, largely synonymous with the process of digestion

Qi vacuity: Insufficient qi manifesting in diminished movement, transformation, and function

Repletion: Excess or fullness, almost always pathological

Seven star hammer: A small hammer with needles embedded in its head used to stimulate acupoints without actually inserting needles

Spirit: The accumulation of qi in the heart which manifests as consciousness, sensory awareness, and mental-emotional function

Stagnation: Non-movement of the qi, lack of free flow, constraint

Supplement: To add to or augment, as in supplementing the qi, blood, yin, or yang

Turbid: The yin, impure, turbid part of food and drink which is sent downward to be excreted as waste

Vacuity: Emptiness or insufficiency, typically of qi, blood, yin, or yang

Vacuity cold: Obvious signs and symptoms of cold due to a lack or insufficiency of yang qi

Vacuity heat: Heat due to hyperactive yang in turn due to insufficient controlling yin

Vessels: The main routes for the distribution of qi and blood, but mainly blood

Viscera: The solid yin organs of Chinese medicine

Yang: In the body, function, movement, activity, transformation

Yang vacuity: Insufficient warming and transforming function giving rise to symptoms of cold in the body

Yin: In the body, substance and nourishment

Yin vacuity: Insufficient yin substance necessary to nourish, control, and counterbalance yang activity

Bibliography

Chinese language sources

Cheng Dan An Zhen Jiu Xuan Ji (Cheng Dan-an's Selected Acupuncture & Moxibustion Works), ed. by Cheng Wei-fen *et al.*, Shanghai Science & Technology Press, Shanghai, 1986

Chu Zhen Zhi Liao Xue (A Study of Acupuncture Treatment), Li Zhong-yu, Sichuan Science & Technology Press, Chengdu, 1990

Fu Ke Lin Chuan Jing Hua (The Clinical Efflorescence of Gynecology), Wang Bu-ru & Wang Qi-ming, Sichuan Science & Technology Press, Chengdu, 1989

Fu Ke Yu Chi (The Jade Ruler of Gynecology), Shen Jin-ao, Shanghai Science & Technology Press, Shanghai, 1983

Fu Ke Zheng Zhi (Gynecological Patterns & Treatments), Sun Jiu-ling, Hebei People's Press, 1983

Gu Fang Miao Yong (Ancient Formulas, Wondrous Uses), Chen Bao-ming & Zhao Jin-xi, Science & Technology Popularization Press, Beijing, 1994

Han Ying Chang Yong Yi Xue Ci Hui (Chinese-English Glossary of Commonly Used Medical Terms), Huang Xiao-kai, People's Health & Hygiene Press, Beijing, 1982

Nan Zhi Bing De Liang Fang Miao Fa (Fine Formulas & Wondrous Methods for Difficult to Treat Diseases), Wu Da-zhen & He Xin-qiao, Chinese National Medicine & Medicinal Press, Beijing, 1992

Nei Ke Bing Liang Fang (Internal Medicine Disease Fine Formulas), He Yuan-lin & Jiang Chang-yuan, Yunnan University Press, Zhongqing, 1991

Qi Nan Za Zheng Jing (Carefully Chosen Curious, Difficult, Miscellaneous Diseases), Huang Bing-yuan, Guangdong Science & Technology Press, Guangzhou, 1996

"A Review of the Chinese Medical Literature on Climacteric Syndrome", Yao Shi-an, *Zhong Yi Za Zhi (Journal of Chinese Medicine)*, #2, 1994, p. 112-114

Shang Hai Lao Zhong Yi Jing Yan Xuan Bian (A Selected Compilation of Shanghai Old Doctors' Experiences), Shanghai Science & Technology Press, Shanghai, 1984

Shi Yong Zhen Jiu Tui Na Zhi Liao Xue (A Study of Practical Acupuncture, Moxibustion & Tui Na Treatments), Xia Zhi-ping, Shanghai College of Chinese Medicine Press, Shanghai, 1990

Tan Zheng Lun (Treatise on Phlegm Conditions), Hou Tian-yin & Wang Chun-hua, People's Army Press, Beijing, 1989

Xian Dai Nan Zhi Bing Zhong Yi Zhen Liao Xue (A Study of the Chinese Medical Diagnosis & Treatment of Modern Difficult to Treat Diseases), Wu Jun-yu & Bai Yong-bo, Chinese Medicine Ancient Books Press, Beijing, 1993

Yi Zong Jin Jian (The Golden Mirror of Ancestral Medicine), Wu Qian *et al.*, People's Health & Hygiene Press, Beijing, 1985

Yu Xue Zheng Zhi (Static Blood Patterns & Treatments), Zhang Xue-wen, Shanxi Science & Technology Press, Xian, 1986

Zhen Jiu Chu Fang Xue (A Study of Acupuncture & Moxibustion Prescriptions), Wang Dai, Beijing Publishing Co., Beijing, 1990

Zhen Jiu Da Cheng (A Great Compendium of Acupuncture & Moxibustion), Yang Ji-zhou, People's Health & Hygiene Press, Beijing, 1983

Zhen Jiu Xue (A Study of Acupuncture & Moxibustion), Qiu Mao-liang *et al.*, Shanghai Science & Technology Press, Shanghai, 1985

Zhen Jiu Yi Xue (An Easy Study of Acupuncture & Moxibustion), Li Shou-xian, People's Health & Hygiene Press, Beijing, 1990

Zhong Guo Min Jian Cao Yao Fang (Chinese Folk Herbal Medicinal Formulas), Liu Guang-rui & Liu Shao-lin, Sichuan Science & Technology Press, Chengdu, 1992

174

Zhong Guo Zhen Jiu Chu Fang Xue (A Study of Chinese Acupuncture & Moxibustion Prescriptions), Xiao Shao-qing, Ningxia People's Press, Yinchuan, 1986

Zhong Guo Zhong Yi Mi Fang Da Quan (A Great Compendium of Chinese National Chinese Medical Secret Formulas), ed. by Hu Zhao-ming, Literary Propagation Publishing Company, Shanghai, 1992

Zhong Yi Bing Yin Bing Ji Xue (A Study of Chinese Medical Disease Causes & Disease Mechanisms), Wu Dun- xu, Shanghai College of TCM Press, Shanghai, 1989

Zhong Yi Fu Ke Zhi Liao Shou Ce (A Handbook of Chinese Medical Gynecological Treatment), Wu Shi-xing & Qi Cheng-lin, Shanxi Science & Technology Press, Xian, 1991

Zhong Yi Hu Li Xue (A Study of Chinese Medical Nursing), Lu Su-ying, People's Health & Hygiene Press, Beijing, 1983

Zhong Yi Lin Chuang Ge Ke (Various Clinical Specialties in Chinese Medicine), Zhang En-qin *et al.*, Shanghai College of TCM Press, Shanghai, 1990

Zhong Yi Ling Yan Fang (Efficacious Chinese Medical Formulas), Lin Bin-zhi, Science & Technology Propagation Press, Beijing, 1991

Zhong Yi Miao Yong Yu Yang Sheng (Chinese Medicine Wondrous Uses & Nourishing Life), Ni Qi-lan, Liberation Army Press, Beijing, 1993

Zhong Yi Nei Ke Lin Chuang Shou Ce (A Clinical Manual of Chinese Medicine Internal Medicine), Xia De-shu, Shanghai Science & Technology Press, Shanghai, 1990

Zhong Yi Nei Ke Xue (The Study of Chinese Medicine Internal Medicine), Zhang Bo-ying *et al.*, Shanghai Science & Technology Press, Shanghai, 1990

Zhong Yi Zi Xue Cong Shu (The Chinese Medicine Self-study Series), Vol. 1, "Gynecology",Yang Yi-ya, Hebei Science & Technology Press, Shijiazhuang, 1987

English language sources

Abnormal Psychology: Current Perspectives, B. L. Alloy, J. Acocella & R. R. Bootzin, McGraw Hill, NY, 1996

A Barefoot Doctor's Manual, revised & enlarged edition, Cloudburst Press, Mayne Isle, 1977

Beyond Prozac, Michael J. Norden, Harper Collins Publishers Inc., NY, 1995

Chinese-English Terminology of Traditional Chinese Medicine, Shuai Xue-zhong *et al.*, Hunan Science & Technology Press, Changsha, 1983

Chinese-English Manual of Common-used Prescriptions in Traditional Chinese Medicine, Ou Ming, ed., Joint Publishing Co., Ltd., Hong Kong, 1989

Chinese Herbal Medicine: Formulas & Strategies, Dan Bensky & Randall Barolet, Eastland Press, Seattle, 1990

Chinese Herbal Medicine: Materia Medica, Dan Bensky & Andrew Gamble, second, revised edition, Eastland Press, Seattle, 1993

Chinese Self-massage, The Easy Way to Health, Fan Ya-li, Blue Poppy Press, Boulder, CO, 1996

A Clinical Guide to Chinese Herbs and Formulae, Cheng Song-yu & Li Fei, Churchill & Livingstone, Edinburgh, 1993

A Clinical Manual of Chinese Herbal Medicine and Acupuncture, Zhou Zhong Ying & Jin Hui De, Churchill Livingstone, Edinburgh, 1997

A Compendium of TCM Patterns & Treatments, Bob Flaws & Daniel Finney, Blue Poppy Press, Boulder, CO, 1996

A Comprehensive Guide to Chinese Herbal Medicine, Chen Ze-lin & Chen Mei-fang, Oriental Healing Arts Institute, Long Beach, CA, 1992

176

Diagnostic and Statistical Manual of Mental Disorders: Fourth Edition, American Psychiatric Association, Washington, DC, 1994

English-Chinese Chinese-English Dictionary of Chinese Medicine, Nigel Wiseman, Hunan Science & Technology Press, Changsha, 1995

Fundamentals of Chinese Acupuncture, Andrew Ellis, Nigel Wiseman & Ken Boss, Paradigm Publications, Brookline, MA, 1988

Fundamentals of Chinese Medicine, Nigel Wiseman & Andrew Ellis, Paradigm Publications, Brookline, MA, 1985

Glossary of Chinese Medical Terms and Acupuncture Points, Nigel Wiseman & Ken Boss, Paradigm Publications, Brookline, MA, 1990

Handbook of Chinese Herbs and Formulas, Him-che Yeung, self-published, LA, 1985

A Handbook of Differential Diagnosis with Key Signs & Symptoms, Therapeutic Principles, and Guiding Prescriptions, Ou-yang Yi, trans. By C.S. Cheung, Harmonious Sunshine Cultural Center, SF, 1987

A Handbook of Menstrual Diseases in Chinese Medicine, Bob Flaws, Blue Poppy Press, Boulder, CO, 1997

Oriental Materia Medica, A Concise Guide, Hong-yen Hsu, Oriental Healing Arts Institute, Long Beach, CA, 1986

Practical Therapeutics of Traditional Chinese Medicine, Yan Wu & Warren Fischer, Paradigm Publications, Brookline, MA, 1997

Practical Traditional Chinese Medicine & Pharmacology: Clinical Experiences, Shang Xian-min *et al.,* New World Press, Beijing, 1990

Practical Traditional Chinese Medicine & Pharmacology: Herbal Formulas, Geng Jun-ying, *et al.,* New World Press, Beijing, 1991

Sacred Sorrow: Embracing and Transforming Depression, John E. Nelson & A. Nelson, Putnam & Sons Publishing, NY, 1996

The English-Chinese Encyclopedia of Practical Traditional Chinese Medicine, Vol. 12: Gynecology, Xuan Jia-sheng, ed., Higher Education Press, Beijing, 1990

The Essential Book of Traditional Chinese Medicine, Vol. 2: Clinical Practice, Liu Yan-chi, trans. by Fang Ting-yu & Chen Lai-di, Columbia University Press, NY, 1988

The Foundations of Chinese Medicine, Giovanni Maciocia, Churchill Livingstone, Edinburgh, 1989

The Merck Manual, 15th edition, ed. by Robert Berkow, Merck Sharp & Dohme Research Laboratories, Rahway, NJ, 1987

The Nanjing Seminars Transcript, Qiu Mao-lian & Su Xu-ming, The Journal of Chinese Medicine, UK, 1985

The Practice of Chinese Medicine, Giovanni Maciocia, Churchill Livingstone, Edinburgh, 1994

"The Role of the Liver in Menstrual Disorders", (Rona) Wang Ru & Brian May, *The Pacific Journal of Oriental Medicine,* Australia, #77, p. 10-17

"A Theoretical and Practical Approach to Psychodynamics Using Traditional Chinese Medicine", Daniel A. Weber, *Pacific Journal of Oriental Medicine,* Mullimbimby, NSW, #10, 1997

The Treatise on the Spleen & Stomach, Li Dong-yuan, trans. by Yang Shou-zhong, Blue Poppy Press, Boulder, CO, 1993

The Treatment of Disease in TCM, Volume 1: Diseases of the Head and Face Including Mental/Emotional Disorders, Philippe Sionneau & Lu Gang, Blue Poppy Press, Boulder, CO, 1996

Traditional Medicine in Contemporary China, Nathan Sivin, University of Michigan, Ann Arbor, 1987

Zang Fu: The Organ Systems of Traditional Chinese Medicine, second edition, Jeremy Ross, Churchill Livingstone, Edinburgh, 1985

General Index

A

abdominal bloating 22, 150
acid regurgitation 52
acne on the face 150
acupuncture, ear 92, 141
acupuncture treatment 63, 86-88,
    90, 92, 139, 144-146, 173
aerobic exercise 104, 105
aging 9, 18, 29, 36, 38, 106, 126
agitation 5, 13, 36, 51, 53, 55, 58,
    74, 107, 108, 132
alcohol 87, 96, 98, 99, 102, 103, 123,
    126, 141
allergies 23, 164
An Mian Pian 81
An Shen Yang Xia Cha 74
anger and frustration 18
anger, easy 51, 55, 89, 108, 110
anger, violent outbursts of 50
anorexia 4, 107
anxiety iii-5, 36, 42, 53, 55, 67, 69,
    74, 80, 100, 107, 113, 114, 122,
    129, 149
apathetic and tired 52
appetite changes 4
appetite, excessive 61, 90
appetite, increased 57, 88
appetite, loss of 3, 22, 50
arms and legs, lack of strength 53
aromatherapy 113, 114, 133-135,
    170
arthritis, rheumatoid 4
asleep, difficulty falling 155
asthma 76

B

Bai Zi Yang Xin Wan 79
basal body temperature 35
belching and burping 50
bipolar disorder 2, 56, 142, 144
births, excessive 106
bleeding, excessive 58
bleeding, heavy or abnormal 21, 75
blood loss, extreme 106

blood, creation of 32, 33
blood pressure, high 5, 74, 111, 131
blood pressure, low 131
breast distention 49, 58, 127, 150
breasts become sore and painful 57
breath, shortness of 76, 153
bruising, easy 12
burn salve, Chinese 124

C

central nervous system, lesions 144
Chai Hu Jia Long Gu Mu Li Wan 69
Chai Hu Shu Gan Wan 70
chest, fullness in the 73
chest oppression 49-52, 90, 126, 127
Ching Wan Hong ointment 124
chocolate 5, 96, 98, 102
chronic fatigue 131
coffee 97, 98, 102, 114
Cognitive Behavioral Therapy 6
cold, aversion to 95
colds 23
concentrating, difficulty 3, 149
concentration, lack of 53, 134
constipation 70, 71, 128, 154
conventional Western therapy 147
coordination, poor 134
cough 76
crying over any little thing 1
crying spells 152
cursing 50
cyclothymia 2

D

Dan Zhi Xiao Yao Wan 69, 76, 77-79
decisions, inability to make 24
delusional disorder 2
depressed mood 2-4
depression, chronic 2, 3, 36, 43, 144
depression, low-grade, chronic 2, 3
depressive episode iv, 1-4, 45, 59,
    137, 138
depressive neurosis 3
diarrhea 70, 71, 149

179

S

SADD 135
schizoaffective disorder 2
schizophrenia 2, 142
seasonal pattern depression 3
seizure disorders 144
selective serotonin re-uptake
    inhibitors 5
self-esteem, low 24
self-loathing 138
seminal emission, involuntary 54-55
seven star hammering 122, 135
sexual activity, excessive 18
sexual energy 98
Shu Gan Wan 70, 72
side effects iv-6, 8, 45, 48, 62, 63, 68,
    84, 114, 136, 141-142, 146, 152, 157
sighing 111, 153
Sivin, Nathan 163, 178
skin and lips were very dry 154
skin cancer 135
skin rash, crusty 47
sleep, loss of 53-55
sleeping, difficulty 1, 88, 155
somnolence 36
sorrow and anxiety 53
speech, delirious 20
speaking incoherently 20
spirit, lassitude of the 53, 54, 62
spots or macules, static 51
SSRI's 5
St Johnswort iv
stomach, upset 5
stomach, uterus, or rectum,
    prolapse of the 82
stools, dry, bound, constipated 50
stools, loose 47, 71, 95, 125, 134
stools, undigested food in the 95
strength, lack of 53, 54, 128, 130,
    134
stress iii, 29-31, 43, 44, 108, 110,
    112, 113, 133, 149, 157
Su Zi Jiang Qi Wan 76
Suan Zao Ren Tang 80
substance dependency 4

suicide, potential for 144
suicide, thoughts of 5, 51, 139, 142
sunlight 134, 135, 138
sweets, craves 57

T

tea, green 130, 131
terminal dribbling 99
thinking and worry 42, 54
thread moxibustion 123
throat, sensation of something stuck
    in his 153
thrombophlebitis 81
thyroid disorder 144
Tian Wang Bu Xin Dan 78
timidity 24, 53, 54
tinnitus 50
To Jing Wan 81
Tong Jing Wan 81
tongue, sores on the tip of 20, 132
tricyclic antidepressants 5

U, V

ulcers, gastric 152
unipolar depression 2
urinary incontinence 12, 99
uterine prolapse 12, 82
vaginal discharge, watery 54
varicosities 81
vegetarian diet 97, 100
violence 5
vision, blurred 5
vomiting 50, 107

W, X, Z

weight gain 58, 88
will, lack of 36
wines, medicinal 126-128, 164
wise woman 39
Wiseman, Nigel 177
Wolfe, Honora Lee 138, 164
worry, thinking and 42, 54
Xiao Chai Hu Wan 71
Xue Fu Zhu Yuan Wan 82
Zoloft iii, 5

OTHER BOOKS ON CHINESE MEDICINE
AVAILABLE FROM BLUE POPPY PRESS
3450 Penrose Place, Suite 110, Boulder, CO 80301
For ordering 1-800-487-9296 PH. 303\447-8372 FAX 303\245-8362

A NEW AMERICAN ACUPUNC-TURE by Mark Seem, ISBN 0-936185-44-9

ACUPOINT POCKET REFERENCE ISBN 0-936185-93-7

ACUPUNCTURE AND MOXI-BUSTION FORMULAS & TREATMENTS by Cheng Dan-an, trans. by Wu Ming, ISBN 0-936185-68-6

ACUTE ABDOMINAL SYN-DROMES: Their Diagnosis & Treatment by Combined Chinese-Western Medicine by Alon Marcus, ISBN 0-936185-31-7

AGING & BLOOD STASIS: A New Approach to TCM Geriatrics by Yan De-xin, ISBN 0-936185-63-5

AIDS & ITS TREATMENT ACCORDING TO TRADITIONAL CHINESE MEDICINE by Huang Bing-shan, trans. by Fu-Di & Bob Flaws, ISBN 0-936185-28-7

BETTER BREAST HEALTH NATURALLY with CHINESE MEDICINE by Honora Lee Wolfe & Bob Flaws ISBN 0-936185-90-2

THE BOOK OF JOOK: Chinese Medicinal Porridges, An Alternative to the Typical Western Breakfast by B. Flaws, ISBN0-936185-60-0

CHINESE MEDICAL PALMIS-TRY: Your Health in Your Hand by Zong Xiao-fan & Gary Liscum, ISBN 0-936185-64-3

CHINESE MEDICINAL TEAS: Simple, Proven, Folk Formulas for Common Diseases & Promoting Health by Zong Xiao-fan & Gary Liscum, ISBN 0-936185-76-7

CHINESE MEDICINAL WINES & ELIXIRS by Bob Flaws, ISBN 0-936185-58-9

CHINESE PEDIATRIC MAS-SAGE THERAPY: *A Parent's & Practitioner's Guide to the Prevention & Treatment of Childhood Illness* by Fan Ya-li, ISBN 0-936185-54-6

CHINESE SELF-MASSAGE THERAPY: The Easy Way to Health by Fan Ya-li ISBN 0-936185-74-0

A COMPENDIUM OF TCM PAT-TERNS & TREATMENTS by Bob Flaws & Daniel Finney, ISBN 0-936185-70-8

CURING ARTHRITIS NATURALLY WITH CHINESE MEDICINE by Douglas Frank & Bob Flaws ISBN 0-936185-87-2

CURING HAY FEVER NATURALLY WITH CHINESE MEDICINE by Bob Flaws, ISBN 0-936185-91-0

CURING INSOMNIA NATURALLY WITH CHINESE MEDICINE by Bob Flaws ISBN 0-936185-85-6

CURING PMS NATURALLY WITH CHINESE MEDICINE by Bob Flaws ISBN 0-936185-85-6

THE DAO OF INCREASING LONGEVITY AND CONSERVING ONE'S LIFE by Anna Lin & Bob Flaws, ISBN 0-936185-24-4

THE DIVINE FARMER'S MATERIA MEDICA (*A Translation of the Shen Nong Ben Cao*) by Yang Shou-zhong ISBN 0-936185-96-1

THE DIVINELY RESPONDING CLASSIC: *A Translation of the Shen Ying Jing from Zhen Jiu Da Cheng*, trans. by Yang Shou-zhong & Liu Feng-ting ISBN 0-936185-55-4

DUI YAO: THE ART OF COMBINING CHINESE HERBAL MEDICINALS by Philippe Sionneau ISBN 0-936185-81-3

ENDOMETRIOSIS, INFERTILITY AND TRADITIONAL CHINESE MEDICINE: A Laywoman's Guide by Bob Flaws ISBN 0-936185-14-7

THE ESSENCE OF LIU FENG-WU'S GYNECOLOGY by Liu Feng-wu, translated by Yang Shou-zhong ISBN 0-936185-88-0

EXTRA TREATISES BASED ON INVESTIGATION & INQUIRY: *A Translation of Zhu Dan-xi's Ge Zhi Yu Lun*, by Yang Shou-zhong & Duan Wu-jin, ISBN 0-936185-53-8

FIRE IN THE VALLEY: TCM Diagnosis & Treatment of Vaginal Diseases ISBN 0-936185-25-2

FLESHING OUT THE BONES: The Importance of Case Histories in Chin. Med. trans. by Chip Chace. ISBN 0-936185-30-9

FU QING-ZHU'S GYNECOLOGY trans. by Yang Shou-zhong and Liu Da-wei, ISBN 0-936185-35-X

FULFILLING THE ESSENCE: A *Handbook of Traditional & Contemporary Treatments for Female Infertility* by Bob Flaws, ISBN 0-936185-48-1

GOLDEN NEEDLE WANG LE-TING: A 20th Century Master's Approach to Acupuncture by Yu Hui-chan and Han Fu-ru, trans. by Shuai Xue-zhong,

A HANDBOOK OF TRADITIONAL CHINESE DERMATOLOGY by Liang Jian-hui, trans. by Zhang & Flaws, ISBN 0-936185-07-4

A HANDBOOK OF TRADITIONAL CHINESE GYNECOLOGY by Zhejiang College of TCM, trans. by Zhang Ting-liang, ISBN 0-936185-06-6 (4th edit.)

A HANDBOOK OF MENSTRUAL DISEASES IN CHINESE MEDICINE by Bob Flaws ISBN 0-936185-82-1

A HANDBOOK of TCM PEDIATRICS by Bob Flaws, ISBN 0-936185-72-4

A HANDBOOK OF TCM UROLOGY & MALE SEXUAL DYSFUNCTION by Anna Lin, OMD, ISBN 0-936185-36-8

THE HEART & ESSENCE OF DAN-XI'S METHODS OF TREATMENT by Xu Dan-xi, trans. by Yang, ISBN 0-926185-49-X

THE HEART TRANSMISSION OF MEDICINE by Liu Yi-ren, trans. by Yang Shou-zhong ISBN 0-936185-83-X

HIGHLIGHTS OF ANCIENT ACUPUNCTURE PRESCRIPTIONS trans. by Wolfe & Crescenz ISBN 0-936185-23-6

**How to Have A HEALTHY PREG-
NANCY, HEALTHY BIRTH with
Chinese Medicine** by Honora Lee Wolfe,
ISBN 0-936185-40-6

**HOW TO WRITE A TCM HER-
BAL FORMULA:** *A Logical Methodology for the Formulation & Administration of Chinese Herbal Medicine in Decoction* by Bob Flaws, ISBN 0-936185-49-X

**IMPERIAL SECRETS OF
HEALTH & LONGEVITY** by Bob
Flaws, ISBN 0-936185-51-1

**KEEPING YOUR CHILD HEAL-
THY WITH CHINESE MEDI-
CINE** by Bob Flaws, ISBN 0-936185-71-6

**Li Dong-yuan's TREATISE ON
THE SPLEEN & STOMACH,** *A
Translation of the Pi Wei Lun* by Yang
Shou-zhong & Li Jian-yong, ISBN 0-936185-41-4

**LOW BACK PAIN: Care & Pre-
vention with Chinese Medicine** by
Douglas Frank, ISBN 0-936185-66-X

**MASTER HUA'S CLASSIC OF
THE CENTRAL VISCERA** by Hua
Tuo, ISBN 0-936185-43-0

THE MEDICAL I CHING: *Oracle
of the Healer Within* by Miki Shima,
OMD, ISBN 0-936185-38-4

**MANAGING MENOPAUSE
NATURALLY with Chinese Medi-
cine** by Honora Lee Wolfe ISBN 0-936185-98-8

**PAO ZHI: Introduction to Process-
ing Chinese Medicinals to Enhance
Their Therapeutic Effect,** by Philippe
Sionneau, ISBN 0-936185-62-1

**PATH OF PREGNANCY, VOL. I,
Gestational Disorders** by Bob Flaws,
ISBN 0-936185-39-2

**PATH OF PREGNANCY, Vol. II,
Postpartum Diseases** by Bob Flaws.
ISBN 0-936185-42-2

**PEDIATRIC BRONCHITIS: Its
Cause, Diagnosis & Treatment Ac-
cording to TCM** trans. by Gao Yu-li and
Bob Flaws, ISBN 0-936185-26-0

**PRINCE WEN HUI'S COOK:
Chinese Dietary Therapy** by Bob
Flaws & Honora Lee Wolfe, ISBN 0-912111-
05-4, $12.95 (Published by Paradigm Press)

**THE PULSE CLASSIC: A Trans-
lation of the *Mai Jing*** by Wang Shu-he,
trans. by Yang Shou-zhong ISBN 0-936185-
75-9

**RECENT TCM RESEARCH
FROM CHINA**, trans. by Charles Chace
& Bob Flaws, ISBN 0-936185-56-2

**THE SECRET OF CHINESE
PULSE DIAGNOSIS** by Bob Flaws,
ISBN 0-936185-67-8

**SEVENTY ESSENTIAL TCM
FORMULAS FOR BEGINNERS**
by Bob Flaws, ISBN 0-936185-59-7

**SHAOLIN SECRET FORMULAS
for Treatment of External Injuries**,
by De Chan, ISBN 0-936185-08-2

**STATEMENTS OF FACT IN
TRADITIONAL CHINESE
MEDICINE** by Bob Flaws, ISBN 0-
936185-52-X,

**STICKING TO THE POINT 1: A
Rational Methodology for the Step
by Step Formulation & Administration of an Acupuncture Treatment** by Bob Flaws ISBN 0-936185-17-1

**STICKING TO THE POINT 2: A
Study of Acupuncture & Moxibus-
tion Formulas and Strategies** by
Bob Flaws ISBN 0-936185-97-X

THE SYSTEMATIC CLASSIC
OF ACUPUNCTURE & MOXI-
BUSTION (*Jia Yi Jing*) by Huang-fu Mi,
trans. by Yang Shou-zhong & Charles Chace,
ISBN 0-936185-29-5

THE TAO OF HEALTHY EATING
ACCORDING TO CHINESE MED-
ICINE by Bob Flaws, ISBN 0-936185-
92-9

THE TREATMENT OF DISEASE
IN TCM, Vol I: Diseases of the Head
& Face Including Mental/Emotional
Disorders by Philippe Sionneau & Lü Gang,
ISBN 0-936185-69-4

THE TREATMENT OF DISEASE
IN TCM, Vol. II: Diseases of the
Eyes, Ears, Nose, & Throat by Sionneau
& Lü, ISBN 0-936185-69-4

THE TREATMENT OF DISEASE,
VOL. III: Diseases of the Mouth,
Lips, Tongue, Teeth & Gums, by
Sionneau & Lü, ISBN 0-936185-79-1

THE TREATMENT OF DISEASE,
VOL VI: Diseases of the Neck, Shoul-
ders, Back, & Limbs, by Philippe Sionneau
& Lü Gang, ISBN 0-936185-89-9

THE TREATMENT OF EXTER-
NAL DISEASES WITH
ACUPUNCTURE & MOXI-
BUSTION by Yan Cui-lan and Zhu Yun-
long, ISBN 0-936185-80-5